NODDING OFF

Also available in the Bloomsbury Sigma series:

NODDING OFF

The Science of Sleep from Cradle to Grave

Alice Gregory

BLOOMSBURY SIGMA

LONDON · OXFORD · NEW YORK · NEW DELHI · SYDNEY

BLOOMSBURY SIGMA
Bloomsbury Publishing Plc
50 Bedford Square, London, WC1B 3DP, UK

BLOOMSBURY, BLOOMSBURY SIGMA and the Bloomsbury Sigma logo
are trademarks of Bloomsbury Publishing Plc

First published in 2018

A catalogue record for this book is available from the British Library

Library of Congress Cataloguing-in-Publication data has been applied for

ISBN: HB: 978-1-4729-4618-8; TPB: 978-1-4729-4617-1;
eBook: 978-1-4729-4615-7

2 4 6 8 10 9 7 5 3 1

Illustrations by Marc Dando

Typeset by Deanta Global Publishing Services, Chennai, India
Printed and bound in Great Britain by CPI Group (UK) Ltd,
Croydon CR0 4YY

Bloomsbury Sigma, Book Thirty-seven

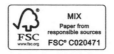

MIX
Paper from
responsible sources
FSC® C020471

To find out more about our authors and books visit www.bloomsbury.com
and sign up for our newsletters

To my parents Jo and Gerry, my husband
The Golden Wolf, and my occasionally
nocturnal children Hector and Orson.
Thank you.

Contents

Note from the Author

Anecdotes are provided to illustrate points made in this book. Apart from those referring to celebrities or scientists, names and details have been altered to protect anonymity. The author is not clinically trained, but is a sleep researcher. Some tips for improving sleep are provided throughout this book. However, before making any alterations to your lifestyle you should talk to your doctor who can consider your personal circumstances and whether changes would be appropriate for you.

Prologue

Bleary-eyed from weeks of partying in sticky-carpeted nightclubs, I slotted myself into the third row of a lecture hall in Oxford. I was attending the last class of term on a course covering mental illness and was preparing for a kip. Sleep was calling and I promised myself that I would study everything on the reading list in exchange for some shut-eye. But I didn't nod off. I listened and hungrily digested every single word.

For an hour, Allison Harvey – then a newly minted lecturer in the Department of Psychology, now a professor at Berkeley, University of California – mesmerised us. Her subject was what I was lacking: sleep. Thinking about it, it seemed odd that despite having spent three years learning about the mind and behaviour, I couldn't recall any other lectures on this topic. And yet Harvey was arguing that our slumber is essential to our waking existence.

She went on to point out that whether we completed our psychology degrees and started a career focusing on child development, educational psychology or mental health, or if we made a living some other way, it would be unwise to underestimate the importance of sleep. This chimed well with my observations of the world. Parents seem desperate for their children to sleep well – not just for their own sanity, but for an almost instinctual fear that if they don't, they won't become the kind, ruddy children they might desire. The notorious teenage lie-ins may be ridiculed and berated by adults, but this behaviour is so common that finding out it is hardwired might come as no surprise. Could it be that attempts to curb it might put our youth at greater risk of flunking exams, having accidents or struggling to regulate their emotions?

For adults, sleeplessness is sometimes feared with such passion that monitoring it interferes with its automaticity. Instead of sleeping, people lie awake worrying about not sleeping. They worry that their work the next day will reflect the mush that they fear their brain will become due to poor sleep. And will they be able to remain temperate when faced with *that colleague*? As loved ones age or become ill, their sleep sometimes deteriorates and we wish them respite in the form of good slumber. Furthermore, Harvey pointed out how little is known about this 'mysterious pastime'. As I have come to realise, even the world's most brilliant sleep researchers still cannot agree on the key functions of sleep, and there is so much more to learn about how it relates to every other aspect of our lives.

That summer I graduated and went to study in Japan for a year. Despite the beauty all around me and the graciousness of the citizens that I met, I was restless living there. I wanted to know more about sleep. So I sent an unsolicited email to Harvey, to ask if I could help with her research from afar. Together we devised a plan for me to hand out questionnaires about sleep to lots of students in Japan and she agreed to do the same in the UK. We would then compare the responses. My husband-to-be was keen to help out, despite the fact that he wasn't a sleep researcher. Together we spent time handing out questionnaires in university dormitories. The results largely suggested that models of insomnia that attribute sleep disturbances to uncontrollable thoughts before we go to sleep might be applicable across these different cultures. While interesting, this research had been conducted on a shoestring and a small scale, so the paper was not going to make a big splash.[1] For me, the main excitement was making a foray into *real* research, together with the realisation that I would be blissfully happy doing this for the rest of my days.

Back in the UK, I started a PhD at King's College London, focusing on social, genetic and developmental psychiatry. Despite the rich and varied topics studied within the institution, there were no sleep experts in my department to guide me, so my desire to focus on this topic seemed somewhat esoteric. I would question colleagues about the data they had collected over the years in long term studies of child development, to see if anyone had asked parents or children about their slumber at any time. I used the data I found, and collected more, to answer questions about whether children who slept poorly were more likely to experience other difficulties in the future, such as anxiety and/or depression.[2] I also looked at the extent to which genes and the environment are important in explaining why sleep problems occur alongside these other difficulties.[3] Were these problems inherited together? I think my key mentors were at times bemused by my passion for this unfamiliar research area. But if they were, they hid it well, and were always overwhelmingly supportive and generous with their time and data.

When I became a lecturer at Goldsmiths, University of London, sleep remained at the forefront of my interests. I ran my own studies to address questions about the relationship between children's thoughts and their sleep.[4] I learned more about how genes influence both our slumber and whether someone functions best in the morning, like a lark, or at night, like an owl.[5] I collaborated with other researchers around the world and was able to share my passion with dedicated students. I would work 6 day weeks and love every second.

Then I hit my 30s and decided to have a baby. This baby would not sleep, which meant that I did not either. Every aspect of my life was affected and all of a sudden every research paper that I had written took on new meaning. Other new parents had an overwhelming interest too, and together we would drift back to this topic of conversation time and time again. I also became more appreciative of how the complexities of life could interfere with the best-intentioned, and informed, prescriptive advice to allow a child to fall asleep alone and without intervention, and how it was perhaps not the desired method for certain parents or was inappropriate for others. I met parent after parent pumped up in the belief that they had found *the* book to resolve their child's sleeplessness. However, more often than not, I watched them appear bereft a few weeks later when a simple sneeze from their baby blew away their carefully balanced sleep formula. Few of the books available seemed to be evidence-based, which made it difficult for parents to understand why they should believe one 'expert' over another. Should they really let their child 'cry it out'? Was it really wrong to nurse their child to sleep when it felt so right? Would the unrelenting sleeplessness never end? Those writing books on children's sleep sometimes declare a magic formula and in instances where they have their own offspring, presumably they sleep beautifully. By contrast, despite my credentials, I did not have all the answers. For one, I was not willing to allow one son, who would occasionally experience frightening seizures during the night, to fall asleep alone. Instead, after he had a spell in hospital, I would spend neurotic hours, semi-delirious, lying on his floor, with his tiny hand in mine, watching his every breath and willing him always to be OK.

That is where the idea for this book was born. I wanted to share my endless passion for the science of sleep, but embed it in the reality of life. Having a baby and experiencing quite dramatic sleep deprivation, and watching sleep patterns develop and change over time, provided the main impetus. However, sleep remains with us and is essential throughout our lives, with each developmental stage providing a different challenge. In childhood and adolescence, sleep deprivation can make children behave as if they have attention deficit hyperactivity disorder (ADHD).* Consequently, youths worldwide are possibly being misdiagnosed with ADHD by clinicians who do not consider their nocturnal habits. When we reach adulthood, our sleep doesn't stop changing and often our demanding working lives dramatically affect it. Some of us must sleep by day and work by night, putting our health in jeopardy. When we reach our retirement years and have time to catch up on sleep, we are presented with further challenges. The eyes of older adults might

---

* This is not to imply that the neurodevelopmental disorder ADHD is not a real condition. Instead it is important to assess the role of sleep in relation to ADHD-like symptoms, as this may be relevant in certain cases.

change so light is filtered in a way that results in their body clock being set less effectively. Even the time of day at which a loved one takes their final breath might be explainable by a constantly evolving science.

Our knowledge of sleep grows daily – and nightly – and only recently have researchers acknowledged the importance of sleep in relation to friendships during adolescence. They have actually brought friends into the laboratory to see how sleeplessness *really* affects our interactions with others.[6] Only in the past few years have we started fully investigating the causes of sleep paralysis, where people find themselves glued to their bed, unable to move.[7] Only now are researchers moving away from considering adult sleep as a solitary pastime and fully embracing the reality that the majority of adults share their bed.[8] But there is so much that we still do not know. Research is progressing quickly and sleeping well is now considered to be at least as important as healthy eating. Every week the media highlights the importance of sleep in connection with something new: the obesity epidemic, cancer, diabetes, Alzheimer's, learning and memory, elite sporting performance, death from accidents, performance at work, creativity, anxiety and depression. But, how can we catch more Zs? Do we really need to go easy on the caffeine and alcohol, but load up on the tart cherry juice and warm milk? Which bits are true and why are we being fed these headlines? For anyone interested in the most underrated third of our lives – this book is for you.

CHAPTER ONE

Sleep 101

I unscrewed the lid of the small brown bottle that had been passed my way. The bottle purportedly contained a substance that would make me feel less anxious. With the precision of a lab technician, I pipetted a few drops of the elixir on to my tongue, unsure of whether it would be a placebo effect if it managed to relax me. The bottle was passed onto the next PhD student, who began to follow suit. Instead she thought better of it and downed the remaining liquid in a single shot. Together we headed to a small seminar room in the decrepit basement of a townhouse in Denmark Hill, London. Outside, ambulance sirens were blaring, coming and going from the large hospital across the way, which didn't help my state of mind. I was about to deliver the first presentation of my PhD work to the brilliant academic staff in my department at King's College London. These folk had been carefully headhunted from around the world and recruited by the university, and they were considered the very best in their fields. Between them they had written thousands of scientific articles that had changed thinking about child development, mental health and genetics. However, none of them knew much about my chosen topic: sleep.

I had practised my presentation feverishly, learning it verbatim. I'd even considered where to pause, smile and tell an off-the-cuff joke. My brain was entirely focused on controlling my anxiety and there was very little left to engage in the moment. The presentation was delivered on autopilot and then the questioning began. I dashed a glance at my potion-gulping comrade to see if she might be willing to ask me a question that would allow me to shine in front of this daunting audience, but her mind appeared to be elsewhere, anticipating her own impending talk.

By contrast, all of the professors seemed typically engaged, with their hands up in eagerness. They were ready to start their line of questioning. Which hand to choose? *Please be kind, please be kind.*

'Yes, Ian?' I selected a professor of genetics, known for his jovial nature.

'So, what exactly do you mean by sleep and why do we bother with it?' he asked.

Having prepared answers about the many complexities of my work, I was somewhat stumped by this seemingly simple question. I garbled my response, burning under the watchful eyes of my mentors, and made a mental note to always start a piece of work on sleep by addressing this question.

What is sleep?

Although we sleep each night, defining it is tricky. What exactly is it? Ask my five- and eight-year-old sons and they'll say it involves 'lying down and doing nothing'. They'll have got the state of relative immobility correct but missed other key features, including that our responsiveness to the world around us is decreased, but it is reversible (we can be woken up). Scientists also point out that before we hit the hay we might also engage in pre-sleep rituals, which vary between species. For most of us, this probably involves brushing our teeth. Location may also help us define sleep. Sleeping people might be found curled up in bed, whereas a bat is more likely to be spied hanging upside down in a cave.

Another simple explanation might involve a switch: one moment we are awake and the next this switch is flicked and we are asleep. When we conk out at night, there *is* a shift in our state, but we are not 'switched off'. There's more to it than that. Our brains and bodies are busy achieving incredible things. There isn't one single change between being awake and in dreamland either, and we exhibit alternations in a range of physiological processes and pass through different stages of sleep. The first stage is so light that if we were woken up, we might not realise we'd dozed off.

So, how can we explain the difference between what we are doing when asleep and when we are playing Sleeping Lions?* Well, the best explanation comes from looking at our physiological state. If someone is hooked up to a sleep monitor, a technique known as 'polysomnography', we'd know exactly when they were no longer faking it. This involves sticking electrodes to various locations on the body and scalp. The electrodes record activity from the brain, eye movements, muscle tone and heart rate. Blood oxygen levels can also be monitored using a painless technique called pulse oximetry, which involves sending light through a body part (such as a fingertip or earlobe). We can't be tricked by someone pretending to be a sleeping lion as having this information means that we are able to work out when someone is truly asleep. If we ask someone how they feel after a night spent playing sleeping lions, as opposed to actually sleeping, their answer would be very different, and it would be easy to discern who had been pretending and who had slept for real. The one who had been pretending would crave sleep and try to make up for what they'd missed.

As to what sleep is *not*, there has been interest in the difference between sleep and general anaesthesia.[1] We even describe doctors 'putting a patient to sleep' when they anaesthetise them before operating so that the patient does not feel any pain. There may be common brain circuits involved in both; however, there are also clear differences. If we tried operating on someone when they were asleep, their movements would be particularly pronounced after the first incision. They would wake up very quickly and scream out in pain. So if sleep is not the same thing as general anaesthesia, what is it? What causes us to fall asleep and wake up from it?

Captain Obvious and the Clock

Two processes appear to control our sleep and wakefulness.[2] One process involves feeling ready to sleep after we've been

---

* A genius game in which small children compete to see who can lie down and be quiet and still for the longest period.

awake for a long time. This might seem as though it is from the school of Captain Obvious. However, it is more complicated beneath the surface. Scientists call this process 'sleep homeostasis' and it refers to our sleep drive.[3] It can be measured by looking at the type of sleep we get. When we are particularly exhausted, and at the beginning of the night, we have more slow-wave sleep. But how exactly does our body know that we've been awake for a long period of time? Scientists are not entirely clear, but among the leading theories is the idea that the longer our brain and the rest of our nervous system has been awake, the greater the accumulation of certain molecules that trigger sleepiness.

One such molecule is adenosine. Adenosine, a by-product of energy metabolism, builds up in the brain of a person who is awake. When caffeine is consumed it blocks the action of adenosine.[4] What is more, following caffeine consumption the body releases adrenaline – sometimes referred to as 'the fight or flight hormone'. This too has less than positive effects on one's ability to fall asleep. It is largely thanks to adenosine that there is a thriving, multiple-billion-dollar coffee industry. Other molecules are important in explaining our sleep drive and there is a lot still to learn. Further discoveries will help to fully solve the puzzle of why it is sometimes so hard to keep our eyes open.

Discussing this mechanism with Daniel Buysse, professor of psychiatry at the University of Pittsburgh, he points out: 'This homeostatic aspect of sleep is unique in that it serves a function that is vital for survival and is partially under voluntary control. However, it can't be replaced. Other functions which are under homeostatic control, partly voluntarily, and essential for survival include eating, drinking and breathing – yet these can be achieved by artificial means such as providing nutrients and fluids intravenously, and using respirators. Sleep is the ONLY homeostatic physiological function that can't be replaced.'

The second process controlling our sleep and wakefulness relates to *when* we fall asleep and wake up. This works like a powerful biological clock, and means that we are more likely to feel tired at night and awake during the day, regardless of when we last slept. There are multiple clocks in different parts of our bodies. In fact, pretty much every cell in our body can have a circadian clock. This means that they are able to provide their own instructions as to when different things should be happening within the cell, such as whether to use energy or repair cell damage. The word 'circadian' comes from the Latin *circa* ('around') and *dies* ('day'). Unsurprisingly then, these processes work on cycles of approximately 24 hours.

The 'master clock' (or the Greenwich clock perhaps) is situated in a small area of the brain called the suprachiasmatic nucleus (SCN). The SCN is located in the hypothalamus, lying deep in our brain. The hypothalamus sits above the optic chiasm – and the latter is important for transmitting signals from the eye to the brain. This 'master clock' is sometimes referred to as a 'conductor', coordinating the clocks throughout the body so they all tick in synchrony, producing a beautiful melody. As to what drives these clocks, in the absence of AA batteries, biology must step up.

In particular, 'clock genes' are key.[5] These give our cells instructions to make certain proteins. This is a complex process. Briefly, certain proteins accumulate over time. Their levels eventually become high enough to enter the nucleus of the cell, or control centre, and switch off the genes that have instructed their very existence. These proteins are either altered or begin to be broken down, and it is only when this happens that the clock genes are able to switch on again and start doing their thing once more. These cycles take around 24 hours, which helps us tick to that beat. Whereas much of our circadian rhythm is controlled from *within* the body, external cues around us are important, and light provides *the* most useful way to get this internal clock locked onto the world around us – as will be discussed later in this book.

Sleep: it's all just a stage

Sleep can be split into different stages. One key distinction is between rapid eye movement (REM) and non-rapid eye movement (NREM) sleep. This probably sounds unexciting – who cares if our eyes are flicking about while we sleep? However, different stages of our slumber are very different beasts. REM sleep is probably the weirdest stage. As the name would suggest, our eyes dart about rapidly, but there are other increases in activity too. Our brain activity is rapid, a bit like when we are awake. Breathing is fast too and we are most likely to dream during REM. From early in life, we stop being able to jerk and twitch and move during this stage of sleep and our body becomes paralysed. This is odd, if we think about it, as everything else seems to be going into overdrive. Perhaps the best explanation is that this paralysis is a survival mechanism. If we were able to act out our dreams who knows where they would take us? A swim in the Thames? A visit to the White House?*

NREM is the term used to describe the rest of our sleep. This is divided into three main parts: N1, N2 and N3. N1 is the lightest stage, where we may still feel half-awake, and N3 is the deepest. Stages are differentiated by electrical activity in the brain, as well as other things such as heart rate, breathing rate and temperature.

When adults fall asleep we enter NREM before REM sleep. Our sleep usually runs in cycles of about 90 minutes throughout the night. Someone who is awake will have brainwaves that have a high frequency (are fast) and are of a small amplitude (not very high). These waves might resemble the rapid little ripples following a tiny pebble hurled into a lake. They are referred to as alpha and beta waves (see figure). As we fall asleep we move into N1 sleep. At this stage, brainwaves tend to have a slightly lower frequency and their amplitude becomes a little larger. These are called theta waves. This stage of sleep is followed by N2, characterised by bursts of electrical activity called sleep spindles, so named because of the shape they produce on an electroencephalogram

---

* In fact, REM sleep behaviour disorder (which will be discussed later) can occur when the paralysis mechanism stops working during REM sleep and there may be vocalisation and/or movement.

(EEG, a technique used to measure brainwaves) printout. During this stage there are other characteristic brain activities referred to as K-complexes. K-complexes are big events of large amplitude on the EEG. They resemble a freak wave, standing out from the others. Our slumber then becomes deeper and during N3, sometimes referred to as deep, delta or slow-wave sleep, we will experience delta and theta waves, which have an even lower frequency and higher amplitude. These waves have more in common with the large rollers encountered far out at sea.

Having reached the deepest stage, we typically move back to N2 before entering our first period of REM sleep. Our sleep cycle is now complete, and we might experience a temporary arousal before we move on to our second cycle of the night and do this over and over again. Not all sleep cycles were created equal – and we tend to spend a greater proportion of them in

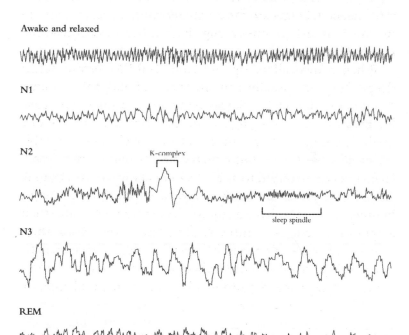

Brain waves characterising different states.

deep sleep during the earliest parts of our slumber compared with the latest. Conversely, we spend a greater proportion of our sleep cycles in REM sleep as the night progresses. The stages and cycles of sleep are referred to as 'sleep architecture'. Structure of sleep is the focus here, just as the structure of buildings is the focus of other types of architecture.

Sleepy brain

What happens in the brain when we fall asleep? Examination of the brain using techniques that look at the electrical activity or activation of particular neuronal structures suggests that it is neither motoring nor idle as we rest. Waking and sleeping, as well as the different stages of sleep, can be thought of as a dance or a balance between the activation and inhibition of discrete brain areas. For example, when we fall asleep an area of the brain called the ventrolateral preoptic (VLPO) nucleus, situated at the front of the hypothalamus, becomes more active. In doing so, brain areas involved in arousal, such as those associated with the ascending reticular activating system (ARAS), are inhibited. The reverse happens when we wake up, with brain areas associated with the ARAS becoming activated and inhibiting areas involved in sleep (such as the VLPO).

As to how brain areas manage to bring about sleep and wakefulness, this is through the release of chemical messengers called neurotransmitters. Areas of the brain controlling the switch between wakefulness and sleep (*i.e.* the VLPO) release neurotransmitters, including gamma-aminobutyric acid, or GABA for short. GABA is an inhibitory neurotransmitter that helps us get some shut-eye by putting the brakes on the wake-promoting neurotransmitters. By contrast, areas of the brain involved in wakefulness (*i.e.* those associated with the ARAS) release neurotransmitters such as orexin, acetylcholine, histamine, dopamine, noradrenaline and serotonin, which send messages throughout the cerebral cortex to keep us awake. The mechanisms are complex and nuanced, but this is the basic gist of what happens in the brain.

Why sleep?

Even the most brilliant scientists don't agree on the matter of
why we sleep, but they agree that it is important. Allan
Rechtschaffen, a professor emeritus at the University of Chicago,
rightly noted: 'If sleep doesn't serve some vital function, it is the
biggest mistake evolution ever made.' So, why do we sleep?

In the 1980s, Rechtschaffen attempted to solve this riddle.
One of his attempts involved depriving animals of sleep. He
placed rats on disks over a pool of water and forced them to
stay awake by revolving the disk if they showed any signs of
sleep. Just as we need to stay alert to navigate the moving
walkway at an airport, the animals needed to be awake to
deal with the rotating disk and if they did not start to walk,
they were plunged into the water.[6] Prolonged sleep deprivation
resulted in a number of physiological changes, such as
problems with thermoregulation, providing clues as to what
sleep might 'keep right' in normal life.

It also became obvious pretty quickly that sleeplessness was
incompatible with life itself. If the rats didn't sleep for two or
three weeks, they died. To distinguish the importance of
different types of sleep, the team of scientists conducted other
studies where they deprived rats of REM sleep alone. By
contrast, they allowed them to enjoy some of the benefits of
NREM sleep. Again, the rats soon died. This time, however,
they typically managed to survive a bit longer, for around
four to six weeks.[*] It may be the case that rats can't survive
long without sleep,[†] but is the same true of people?

---

[*] It must have been agonising to have been a researcher involved in
this type of study, as en route to death the animals became
progressively skeletal, cold and ulcerated. Although seminal in the
field of sleep research, it is unlikely that experiments of this type
would be conducted today. There are strict regulations in place to
minimise the suffering of animals involved in research.

[†] Other explanations have been proposed for the results of the
experiments, such as the role of stress or circadian disruption.
However, the authors of the original paper consider them unlikely.

This question is easier to ask than answer. Fortunately, there is no ethics committee in the world that would allow studies aimed at depriving participants of sleep to the extent that they are at risk of serious harm. Instead, we can draw inferences from naturally occurring sleeplessness. A dramatic example includes people suffering from the rare genetic disease fatal familial insomnia (FFI). People with this disease can miss out on sleep and die within an average of 18 months of symptoms developing.[7] This disorder is an example of a prion disease, whereby abnormal proteins build up in the brain, causing damage. FFI attacks the thalamus, which is a part of the brain that is essential in sleep–wake cycles. Those with this disorder have unusual sleep patterns, including a reduction in sleep length and a disorganisation and deterioration of sleep stages. Eventually there can be a total inability to sleep. While the combination of sleeplessness and death is sometimes used to suggest that the former has caused the latter, this shouldn't be assumed. Instead, other features of this devastating degenerative disease could bring about the end of life – and symptoms of FFI span more than just insomnia, including dementia, as well as difficulties with speech, swallowing and temperature regulation.

Historical cases of total and prolonged sleep deprivation have also provided information about the importance of our slumber.* Take Randy Gardner for example.[8] He was a high-school student who, as part of a scientific study, was deprived of sleep for 264 hours in the 1960s – without even so much as a coffee or other stimulants to keep him going. He was reported to have suffered a range of problems during his sleep deprivation – including a lack of coordination, irritability and delusions.

Then, around the time I was submitting my PhD in 2004, there was a reality TV show that involved depriving 10 participants of sleep over the course of a week as they

---

* These studies do not necessarily prevent all sleep as it is difficult to prevent microsleeps from occurring, for example.

competed for up to £100,000 in prize money. It seemed striking that such an experiment was permitted in the name of entertainment. I am not sure it would still be allowed in the name of science – especially since the findings from the original rat studies are so stark and well known. The winner of the programme, Clare, endured severe sleep deprivation for more than seven days. She managed to stay awake by repeatedly singing songs in her head and playing blinking games. The effects of sleep deprivation on the contestants were very visible and somewhat similar to those experienced by Gardner. Tempers frayed. Hallucinations occurred and one contestant believed that he was the prime minister of Australia. It is clear that we need sleep and sleep deprivation leads to an inability to control emotions, hallucinations and delusions. But *why* is sleep so critical to us?

Theories of sleep

One of the main theories of sleep is that we do it to save energy or to avoid danger – and these are sometimes referred to as 'evolutionary theories'. These theories have merit, and might be a piece of the puzzle, but can they *fully* explain why we sleep? Take the energy-saving hypothesis. Here it is proposed that we use less energy when we are asleep. This is due to our decreased body temperature and other physiological changes associated with sleep, such as a lower metabolic rate during NREM sleep. Support for this theory comes from looking at an animal's size and the amount of sleep they need. On the whole, smaller animals, which have a higher metabolic rate and use up energy more quickly, sleep for longer periods. Golden hamsters might sleep for around 14.3 hours a day, whereas giraffes probably need more like 1.9 hours a day.[9] Of course the situation is not entirely clear cut and, despite being small, guinea pigs sleep for around 9.4 hours a day, whereas the much bigger tiger gets more like 15.8 hours a day.

Advocates of the energy-saving hypothesis sometimes draw an analogy with hibernating animals. They manage to save energy throughout the winter by slowing their metabolism greatly and dropping their body temperature to as low as -2.9°C.[10] But sleep is not hibernation – the energy saving we do while we sleep does not appear to amount to much. Do you know how much energy we save by sleeping for a night rather than staying awake? It's been estimated at just 134 calories.[11] That's less than my favourite chocolate bar, consumed on the way home after a long day in the office. Why wouldn't we save *more* calories if sleep's main function is to save energy? Perhaps because energy is required for the essential physiological processes occurring while we sleep. Moreover, when we start to think about the different stages of sleep this theory makes even less sense. REM sleep, which involves wake-like brain activity, does not appear to save *any* energy at all compared with being awake. Forget the chocolate bar, the energy saving doesn't even justify consumption of an extra celery stick.

Finally, it's been found that some animals are particularly unlikely to save energy when asleep – such as dolphins who sleep half a brain at a time and can continue to move about.[12] Yes, dolphins (and certain other sea animals such as whales and porpoises, and occasionally birds too, for that matter) sleep in a peculiar way. When they are ready to catch some Zs, just one hemisphere of their brain sinks into sleep mode – interestingly, deep, slow-wave sleep only, rather than REM sleep. The other hemisphere retains some level of vigilance to the surrounding world. Dolphins also shut just one eye (usually the one on the opposite side to the sleeping hemisphere). These animals swap hemispheres too, so that both sides of the brain can benefit from sleep. As to why this occurs, it has been proposed that this allows these animals to come to the surface to breathe, to keep track of what is going on in the environment and to generate heat. So, it would seem that dolphins and some other creatures can keep moving while half of their brain stays awake. They are therefore unlikely to sleep in such a way that saves much energy, yet they still sleep. It would seem there might be other reasons for doing so. Rather than seeing sleep as a method of saving energy, it has been argued more convincingly that different behavioural states allow for energy to be allocated optimally to vital biological processes.[13]

As for avoiding danger, the idea here is that if tucked up in bed, we are less likely to be getting up to mischief. The same goes for other animals, who attempt to snuggle down out of harm's way when they are ready for sleep. But does this *really* make sense? Diurnal animals such as you and I sleep at the creepiest time, when our surroundings are at their darkest.* When asleep we lose vigilance so are surely more vulnerable compared to when we are awake. The dangers posed by predators are increased – and we're at greater risk of being on the receiving end of all kinds of heinous crimes. I myself have been a victim of being photographed during slumber: mid-snore, double chin and drool!

As for the theories that make more sense, it seems that getting some Zs gives the brain and body a chance to restore themselves. We do know that sleep allows the body a special opportunity to make certain hormones at night. During deep sleep, the release of growth hormone peaks. This is important for cell reproduction, allowing our bodies to replace damaged or dying cells, and letting us grow and change. Sleep allows us to retune and restore the fine balance of the physiological processes in the body.

One of the more recent restoration theories proposes that we sleep because it allows the brain to take a 'shower' and we wash away the toxins that have accumulated during the day.[14] The idea here is that toxins build up in the brain while we're awake. These come in different forms, but one that has been well studied is beta amyloid – amino acids centrally involved in the development of Alzheimer's disease. When it comes to getting some shut-eye, certain brain cells shrink, allowing more space for fluid to remove these toxins.

---

* A diurnal lifestyle involves being active during the day and asleep at night.

A further theory of sleep proposes that it is key for information and memory processing.[15] It's not that we learn new information during our sleep, but rather that we consolidate what we have learnt during the day. Some of us might relate to that feeling of going to bed with a fuzzy brain when revising for an exam, unsure of what's been learnt and how to integrate this knowledge. We might then wake up with the filing in our brains completed, with everything neatly stored away where it should be and ready to be regurgitated at the drop of a hat.

While some students prioritise getting forty winks during periods of exam revision, others may be taken by the appeal of the 'all-nighter'. Be warned though! This can backfire and students who revise night after night for exams can struggle with multiple aspects of their well-being. The evidence is clear that disregard for sleep is not a good way forward; however, people cope in different ways. Many of us know that jammy classmate who enjoyed a lot of raucous fun, before acing exams following a stint of around the clock studying; or the one who claims to do their best work under pressure at 3 a.m. As with so many things in life, individual differences shouldn't be ignored.

As well as helping us to learn endless facts for exams, sleep is important for other types of memory and learning too. Dr Dan Denis, a postdoctoral researcher on sleep and memory at Harvard Medical School and a collaborator of mine, says: 'There is some great research showing that if you have participants do a creative thinking task after sleep they are more creative. What's more they are better able to decide which idea is the most creative from a list of ideas they made before going to sleep'. This might help to explain why some people have had the experience of waking up with that 'eureka' feeling, where a problem is resolved after a good night's sleep. The lucky few have found the solution to the most incredible problems, including Mendeleev consolidating his ideas for the periodic table of chemical elements following sleep.[16] Legend has it, he had been struggling for some time to classify the elements in the table, but woke up with the problem resolved – he had dreamt the solution. In contrast, for many of us, a eureka feeling might involve something more mundane such as resolving what to cook for dinner. Denis goes on to point out that sleep enhances procedural (motor skills), declarative (e.g. memories of explicit events) and emotional memories too.

So how are learning and memory consolidated during the night? Multiple processes are likely to be important. When we learn, we are left with a weak memory of what we have been exposed to, which then needs to be made more stable and enduring. Denis elaborates: 'The brain is also able to prioritise which memories are consolidated during sleep. It appears to prioritise weakly encoded memories (so you could imagine the brain thinking "oh this memory isn't very well formed, it should be strengthened during sleep") and memories that are of future relevance (the brain prioritises what it thinks is most important to remember).'

It is believed that sleep is involved in memory consolidation by reactivating newly formed memory representations. Denis goes on to say: 'This reactivation aids in the redistribution of memories from short-term storage in a part of the brain called the hippocampus into longer-term storage in areas of the cortex. This reactivation process is thought to occur during periods of non-REM sleep. This aspect of sleep has been shown to benefit both declarative or episodic memory (such as that of facts and knowledge), and procedural memory (our memory of how to do things, such as to walk or ride a bike). Following reactivation during non-REM sleep, REM sleep is thought to be important in stabilising reactivated memories to ensure they remain in long-term storage, integrated with other relevant memories. There is also evidence that highly emotional memories undergo extra processing during REM sleep periods.' He concludes that 'whilst the full picture isn't clear yet, research shows that all stages of sleep are important in memory consolidation'.

When we learn and remember, not only do we need to establish and strengthen connections between brain cells, but we need to eliminate some paths too. Out with the old to make space for the new. The synaptic homeostasis theory of sleep proposes that during the day we are bombarded with information and that our brains build new networks as a result.[17] This could potentially overwhelm and prevent us from being able to absorb new information. In order to cope with this, sleep arrives, providing respite for the brain and allowing rebalancing of neurons' synaptic inputs. Indeed, during deep sleep, pathways that are not so important are believed to be weakened, taking pressure off the brain. So, is it that pathways in the brain are strengthened when we sleep or are they eliminated? The answer is probably both.

Another theory – which has been used to explain the intricate links between sleep and mental health – focuses on emotional recalibration. This theory was proposed by the scientist Matthew Walker, professor of neuroscience and psychology at the University of California, Berkeley. Together with colleagues, he suggested that sleep, and particularly REM sleep, somehow provides 'overnight therapy'.[18]

In a BBC article, Walker was reported as noting that our first memories are typically of events involving great emotions, but over time such memories no longer elicit the same emotional reaction.[19] The 'horror' of being left alone in a cot will not leave us frightened or tearful decades later. This has been explained as REM sleep allowing us to go over events that have occurred and uncouple them from the emotional component. The mechanisms by which this occurs are likely to be complex. However, biological characteristics of REM sleep – such as the very low levels of noradrenaline, related to anxiety and stress, in our brains – allow emotional experiences to be reactivated and stored as memories, while at the same time reducing the emotional arousal associated with the original event.[20] This all means that we can learn and move forward without being too distressed to cope with our continuing lives.

Sleep: what's it all about?

The reasons for sleep are still baffling and causing debate, but it is clear that slumber is important for pretty much every area of our physical and mental functioning. Walker recently pointed out that every single system in our body is aided by sleep – including those related to our immunity, reproduction, metabolism, cardiovascular functioning and ability to control our body temperature.[19] 'Is there anything that isn't improved by sleep, or impaired by sleep deprivation?' he wondered. 'The answer is no.' When I discuss this with Dr Michael Grandner, director of sleep and health research at the University of Arizona College of Medicine, he elaborates: '"What is the function of sleep?" is like asking "what is the function of being awake?". There is no one function and at the end of the day our biology requires both.' When I think back to the behaviour displayed by the participants of that TV show who were sleep deprived for an entire week, the emotional outbursts, hallucination and delusions make sense. Sleep is essential for our waking lives.

Overall, it seems that there are some universal functions of sleep that are common across all animals, but there are also differences in sleep across species and individuals. Could there also be a malleable role of sleep that is tailored to the individual? Is sleep the ultimate personal assistant pandering to our every need, restocking our cupboards and shelves when they are beginning to look empty, filing the unrelenting paperwork generated during the day and preparing for what is to come? At different stages of our lives the demands made on our internal assistant differ. Sleep in youth plays an important role in brain maturation,[21] whereas at the other end of life, it is likely to be more important for preventing brain deterioration.[22] Perhaps this also explains some of the inconsistencies in sleep between different animals.[23] Indeed, it has been pointed out by Jerome Siegel, Professor of Psychiatry and Biobehavioural Sciences at the University of California, Los Angeles, that there are multiple differences between animals in terms of their sleep. For example, stop a rat from sleeping by making it walk on a rotating disk over water and it will quickly die. If we do the same to a pigeon, it will cheat by leaning on the wall to get some Zs or perhaps grab some unihemisphere sleep and it will keep on strolling. Lions enjoy sleep fit for a king – deep and protracted; whereas

the long, lean giraffe has to make do with light and brief
sleep. Check out the night-time erections of men and
armadillos and you'll see they occur at quite different stages
of sleep, men during REM and armadillos during non-REM.

What's in a dream?

Before concluding this chapter, we need to talk about dreams.
It would leave things incomplete to present theories of sleep
without considering why we dream. Brilliant artists, authors
and my five-year-old son alike all find dreams endlessly
interesting. They provide screenwriters with the ultimate tool.
No fan of 1980s TV series *Dallas* could forget the sight of
Bobby Ewing in the shower after he was killed off and brought
back, and the events of the passing year were declared 'a dream'.
But, amazingly, those with the greatest interest in sleep (sleep
researchers) often steer away from this topic. This is, in part,
because dreams are so difficult to study scientifically. After all,
the only way we can find out about the subjective experience
of dreaming is to ask people about their dreams when they are
awake.

Assuming that Roald Dahl was incorrect, and dreams are
not a result of giants blowing them into our bedrooms at
night,[24] why do we dream? To summarise a few of the theories
that have gained the most attention, why not start with Freud.
Freud suggested that dreams provide us with clues as to what
is going on in the 'unconscious mind'. He proposed that this
is the part of our mind that we may not be aware of and
which is full of symbols. He suggested that our dreams
sometimes constitute a way of fulfilling our hidden desires
and wishes, and dreams were analysed in an attempt to learn
more about the unconscious mind.

However, many scientists struggle with Freud, as his theories
are not based on systematic experimentation on representative
samples. As a scientist you are taught to collect data from enough
people to be able to test a theory. However, Freud appeared to
base most of his ideas upon his own experiences and musings,
and those of his patients. It is unclear how applicable these ideas

are to the wider population around us. It also appears to be difficult, if not impossible, to test some of his theories.

Other theories have focused on the emotional significance of dreams. It has been proposed that dreams help us to process and deal with our emotions.[25] This can help to explain why 'sleeping on it' can be helpful in allowing us to deal with negative emotions.

Another model, the activation–synthesis model of dreaming, was put forward by Allan Hobson, a now emeritus professor of psychiatry at Harvard Medical School. This model states that different areas of the brain are activated during REM sleep.[26] These can include brain areas involved in different functions, such as emotions and memories. This can result in rather nonspecific brain activity. The idea here is that the brain then tries to make sense of this activity (or rather synthesises it). This results in what we experience as dreams and can perhaps help to explain why dreams are so often peculiar. This theory is unpopular among those who want dreams to have a deeper meaning.

Subsequently, Hobson proposed a theory of 'protoconsciousness'. Here, dreaming is considered useful in providing a virtual–reality model of the world, which can allow us to develop our skills of higher consciousness, including self-awareness and the ability to reflect on our own thought processes.[27]

Almost 20 years ago, in a dusty basement in Denmark Hill, Ian, professor of genetics, asked me: 'So, what exactly do you mean by sleep, and why do we bother with it?' It might have taken me almost two decades to get back to him, but that's not too bad, given the complexities of these issues. After all, even the world's greatest scientists disagree on how best to answer these questions. The science of sleep is constantly evolving and another 20 years from now my answer to Ian will be much richer than it is today.

CHAPTER TWO

Sleeping Like a Baby: Sleep in the First Years of Life

Infants (4–12 months) recommended 12–16 hours of sleep per 24 hours
Toddlers (1–2 years) recommended 11–14 hours of sleep per 24 hours[1,]*

My husband's fixed smile might have fooled the lady poking my belly, but to my trained eye, it was more grimace-like. The waiting game was unbearable. And there was our baby, motionless, except for a slight sway, attributable to the liquor of his private pool. My stare turned to the sonographer whose stony face was unflinching while pushing, poking, clicking and measuring. As she passed me a tissue to wipe the gunk off my belly, a smile cracked through. 'I think the baby's sleeping! That bodes well.' And there I could witness my beautiful son. I took some time to process my relief that the scan had revealed no problems and to soak up the delight in having seen our baby. But then the sonographer's comment about sleep came back to me. Wasn't it interesting that straight after checking the vital measurements of our child she had thought about his sleep? Was my area of expertise noted in my file perhaps? Maybe, maybe not, but talk of the baby sleeping in utero had already been raised by a number of people. And this was discussed even more relentlessly once

---

* Sleep requirements differ between people. Recommendations provided in the chapters on children and adolescents (aged 0–18) are based on experts reviewing research on sleep duration and health. These recommendations have been endorsed by the American Academy of Pediatrics and the Sleep Research Society. However, some experts think that we do not yet have enough data to make precise recommendations of this type.

our baby was born. 'How does he sleep?' was often the first
question I was asked upon introducing him to friends,
relatives and even strangers. But why this fascination with
infants' sleep?

We are often oblivious to the sleeping patterns of our
babies while they're in the womb. It's only once they're born
that it becomes an obsession and parents so often trade their
own sleep for that of their babies. For me, by the time I
became a mother, I'd been studying sleep as a student and
professionally for almost 10 years – and at the age of 32, the
equivalent of over 10 whole years of my life had been spent
fast asleep. But witnessing this enigmatic process develop in
my newborn son, and eventually trying to marshal when and
for how long he did it, was a revelation to me. Babies sleep a
lot and they also sleep very differently from adults. Careful
studies of young infants have revealed how sleep is tailored to
this stage of life, while also giving clues as to its elusive overall
functions.

So, yes, newborn babies sleep a lot – even if for a new
parent it might not always feel that way. Their dedication to
this is amazing. Newborn babies can easily sleep for more
than 17 hours a day. By the time they reach 4–12 months they
often spend around 12–16 hours a day sleeping. What a long
time to spend asleep! Wouldn't it be better for a baby to be
wide awake and learning from the surrounding world instead?
But sleep and learning are not mutually exclusive. In fact, in
addition to consolidating memories, it's been found that
infants can actually learn new information while asleep.
Indeed, if you were to play sleeping babies a tune and then
blow gently into their eyes, upon hearing the music they
would soon come to expect the air and scrunch up their
eyelids.[2]

The challenge for most parents is not the amount of time
their babies sleep, but when they sleep. During my pregnancy
I remember reading an article stating that 'sleep consolidation
occurs during the first six months of life and becomes more
concentrated during the night'. What this actually meant was
that as a new parent I would probably get no undisturbed

sleep for six whole months: **NO UNDISTURBED SLEEP FOR SIX WHOLE MONTHS!** And for many, the initial six months may represent only the beginning of the all-night party. A huge international study supporting this idea involved questioning almost 30,000 parents about the sleep of their babies and toddlers. It was found that in their first couple of months, babies woke up around twice a night.[3] While this might be expected, it was perhaps more sobering that even two- to three-year-olds still tended to wake up about once at night. The study confirmed what seasoned parents already know and provided scientific support for the marathon of sleep disturbance that new parents embark on.

Why keep waking?

As to why infants wake during the night, this is probably easiest to understand by thinking back to Captain Obvious and the Clock (see Chapter 1). These processes work quite differently in infants than they do in adults. Take for example Captain Obvious, which is the general idea that the longer we stay awake the greater our sleep drive. The neurotransmitter systems involved in this process are underdeveloped at birth, so this does not work in the same way as it does later in life. Adults need to stay awake for much longer periods than infants to feel tired enough to drop off. Three to four hours into the day, just when adults are getting going, a baby may be coasting towards a nap.[4]

However, the circadian clock is probably causing even bigger problems, and is the reason why young babies don't start out showing day-and-night the respect it deserves. At birth, the clock is not yet developed and so is not ticking to a 24-hour beat.[5] A new baby's wake and sleep pattern is not yet on a 24-hour cycle. Just as their visual systems and language skills need time to develop, so do their body clocks, which need to latch on to the world around them. As a result, somewhat excruciatingly for parents, it's equally likely that sleep will occur during the day or night. In the first three months of life, the brain develops greatly and the internal clock begins to synchronise with day and night. By three months things are looking up and most sleep happens at night – although it continues to remain fragmented for some time.

While much of the development is automatic, parents can help. As a baby develops, exposure to light is the most useful way to get this internal clock locked on to the world. Therefore, joining buggy-fit and getting babies out and about during the day, and investing in a blackout blind and putting them in darkness at night, is a good way to help them begin to establish the pattern of sleeping that most people desire. Other things help too. While newborn babies produce very little of their own darkness hormone melatonin, the ticking of a mother's biological clock means that evening and night breastfeeds contain more melatonin. This hormone might provide the infant with a clue that it is time to fall asleep.[6] Melatonin is released from the pineal gland in the brain when light levels are low and can tell us that it is time to fall asleep. If we think back to the master clock in the suprachiasmatic nucleus or SCN discussed earlier – it is this that controls melatonin production. Melatonin is often thought of as the sleep hormone, but that is not accurate as it can make some animals spring into action. The key feature of melatonin is that it is released at dusk rather than when we want to go to sleep, so if you are a nocturnal animal it may signal that it's time to wake up. For the likes of you and I, assuming you are not a vampire, it is more likely to make us feel sleepy. Melatonin is therefore perhaps best referred to as the 'darkness hormone'. It tells a creature to do what it should be doing at night.

By six months, the body clock usually works pretty well and ticks away happily until adolescence, at which point sleep changes so dramatically that we could be forgiven for thinking that the battery might need replacing.

As well as sleep timing, sleep stages in infants are quite different from those experienced by adults. In fact, they're so distinct that the stages are given different names. Something approximating REM sleep is known as 'active sleep' in babies younger than six months. It has this name because the babies are jerky and twitchy during this stage of sleep. They breathe quickly and irregularly and make little movements and noises.

From early on in life babies may also grin during this stage of sleep – something that is particularly exciting, as their smiles may not yet have emerged during their waking lives. When I discuss this with my colleague at Goldsmiths, University of London, Dr Caspar Addyman, expert on babies' laughter and author of *The Laughing Baby*, he tells me: 'If one function of sleep is to regulate emotion, then we should not be too surprised if very small babies are experiencing emotions in their sleep. Even newborn babies experience emotions. In fact, using high-definition ultrasound, a team of researchers at the University of Durham have found that genuine smiles and even practice laughter are already seen in the womb when the baby is in a state not unlike early "active sleep".'

The activity during this stage of sleep is quite different from the paralysis experienced by adults. In adults, the brainstem (the part of the brain connected with the spinal cord) blocks nerve impulses going to the muscles during REM sleep, causing a state of paralysis that stops us acting out our dreams. This mechanism is not yet working fully in newborn babies and is not matured until 6–12 months of age.[7] Interestingly, the development of this paralysis mechanism coincides with a baby's ability to get up to mischief. It keeps them safe when they are asleep at a time when their mobility has stepped up a gear and they have the potential to get into danger.

In contrast, NREM sleep in babies is known as 'quiet sleep', during which they are still. Before six months, NREM sleep can't be fully split into the stages seen so clearly later in life. For example, 'sleep spindles' (brief little bursts of electrical activity, characteristic of N2 sleep, mentioned in Chapter 1) don't develop until an infant is a couple of months old, the stage at which they are typically cooing and gurgling. Slow-wave sleep, characteristic of N3 sleep, which is used to provide information about sleep homeostasis (or Captain Obvious), emerges only at about three months – the same stage of life when smiles are often abundant. Even later, at about six months, when babies are typically learning to crawl, K–complexes, another electrical hallmark of N2 sleep, are fully developed.

Finally, even the *order* in which sleep stages are experienced differs between newborns and older humans. Instead of entering NREM before REM, babies younger than three months have a reversed pattern starting with active REM–like sleep and only later moving on to quiet NREM sleep.[4] They're reading the book back to front.

Part of the reason that sleep looks so different may well be attributable to the different stages serving different functions. The fact that newborn babies spend approximately 50 per cent of their sleep in a REM–like state, whereas this is just 25 per cent by the age of two, provides us with important clues. Could it be that this type of sleep is particularly important for the developing brain?[8] This makes sense given that REM–like sleep is most abundant during the life stages when brain development is at its fastest. REM sleep is greatest when the brain is most 'plastic' – or amenable to lasting change – and when it is forming connections at formidable rates, never to be reached again.

One area that REM may facilitate is the functional development of the visual system.[9] Vision is an important sense to which a huge proportion of our brain is devoted. During the earliest stages of life, babies need to make sense of the visual information in the world around them. Just think about what an accomplishment that is. They take a mass of visual stimuli – a bombardment of photons colliding with their immature retinas – and create meaning out of it. Gradually, they learn to focus on what is important and to coordinate their eyes, so that they track objects and perceive depth. Early visual experiences occur while the infant is awake. However, the effects of these experiences on the brain – when connections between neurons and between brain regions are strengthened, weakened or even eliminated – may well happen offline during REM–like sleep.

Problems in the past?

While suffering the challenges of night waking, parents of young infants can be tormented further by the way their children's sleep changes from one night to the next. Night-to-night variation can make the weather look like a paragon of stability. When a parent joyously declares that their young infant has started 'sleeping through the night',* we have to wonder whether it will last. One night of uninterrupted sleep doesn't mean that disturbed nights are a thing of the past, just as a ray of sunshine in March doesn't forecast a glorious summer.

Anything that can cause pain or discomfort can affect infant sleep. This translates to potentially problematic sleep for any child who has an upset stomach, headache, slight cold, earache, or arm ache from an injection, plus any kid with a wonky nappy, a Babygro that was washed with (or perhaps without) fabric conditioner, or who is placed in a room that's a little too hot or cold for their liking. Thinking about it in that way, it seems a miracle that babies ever sleep. Just as our eating habits change day-to-day depending on our activity, we shouldn't necessarily expect our children's sleep quality to remain identical each night.

Then there are child-by-child differences. Certain parents can't help themselves declaring that their child 'slept through the night' from four weeks old (perhaps they should read *How to Win Friends and Influence People*?[10]). When I became a parent, I met a mother, Saskia. She would arrive for coffee with freshly washed hair and a breezy confidence about her new found parenting skills. She was always pleased to share her successes with me and once declared that her daughter had

---

* The definition of 'sleeping through the night' differs dramatically between parents. Arousals during the night are normal, but many fall back to sleep straight away without much awareness of this. Furthermore, one parent may consider five consecutive hours as a full night, whereas another may expect many more consecutive hours before they consider their child to be 'sleeping through the night'.

been sleeping through the night since she was four weeks old. Saskia claimed to be a 'natural parent'. In contrast, another friend, Lucy, would arrive at get-togethers with coffee stains down her shirt. Lucy revealed tearfully that her life had become chaotic and she was struggling with her baby's sleep and felt it was testing her sanity. While some of these reported differences between offspring may reflect interpretation or an enthusiasm for bragging, others may be genuine. After all, every person is unique. Whereas some children spend their time hatching genius plans to stay awake late, others can be spied trying to slope off to sleep unnoticed. I still don't know what happened in the TV show *Twin Peaks*, broadcast in the early 1990s, due to my total inability (retained to this day) to stay awake late.

Genetic and environmental differences

One way that I have tried to understand differences between people in terms of their sleep, is to look at huge numbers of twins. Even if you know nothing about twin research, you will have noticed that twins come in two flavours.[11] There are those who look impossibly alike, which can lead to all kinds of confusion and high jinks. Then there are the others who look so dissimilar you might fail to realise they are even related. George and Fred Weasley from *Harry Potter* are a good example of the former, with Arnold Schwarzenegger and Danny DeVito in the film *Twins* a somewhat far-fetched example of the latter.

Studying these twins can tell us something about how important genes are in explaining differences between people. The logic goes like this: identical twins are genetic clones of one another. They both originate from the same single fertilised egg. They also often share the same environment in lots of ways: they have the same parents and usually live in the same house in the same neighbourhood. As they grow older they often go to the same school.

Then there are non-identical twins who are also alike for the same reasons (because of their genes and because of things in their environment). The only difference is that they are not genetic clones of one another. Instead, they are the result of two eggs fertilised by different sperm. They have genes that make them different from one another (and like any other full-sibling pairs share just 50 per cent of their segregating genes, or rather those genes that explain differences between people).

So, when we see that identical twins' sleeping patterns are more similar than non-identical twins' (as we often do) we draw the conclusion that genes are playing a role. An example of work of this type came from a team of researchers based at University College London.[12] They asked the parents of twins aged 15 months old all about their sleep. Parents' responses suggested that twins within a family had almost identical bedtimes, regardless of whether they were identical or non-identical twins. However, their responses also indicated that identical twins were more similar to one another than non-identical twins for all other aspects of sleep assessed. These included the time they woke up, their night-time sleep duration, the duration of their naps and their sleep disturbances. From this information the researchers concluded that, to varying extents, genes influenced all of these things.*

So what should we do with the information that one baby may sleep better than another partly because of their genes? Celebrate! New parents can be suffocated with guilt. They wonder: 'Is my child's sleeplessness due to over- or under-feeding? Poor sleep practices? Parental incompetence?' Certainly, my friend Lucy revealed concerns like these and blamed herself endlessly when her baby would not sleep. Hopefully, knowing that the genes we are born with have some influence on our sleep is one piece of information that

---

* In this study, genes did not help to explain variation in bedtime, but influenced other aspects of sleep (explaining from 26 per cent to 40 per cent of the variance). Heritability is a population statistic, meaning that estimates may be different when studying other populations.

will help to alleviate anxiety. If one child is awake more than their peers, then perhaps that's just the way they are wired. So when accosted by someone like Saskia – regaling gleefully that their four-week-old child sleeps all night, every night – we should know that this is unlikely to reflect parental competence. Lucy and Saskia may have had very different starting points with their children.

But does the finding that genes influence the way we sleep also mean that techniques can't be used to improve sleep? If our grandparents, parents and children are all poor sleepers, could nights spent lying awake be our destiny? Not necessarily. In fact, one of the first lessons a student of behavioural genetics learns is that just because genes influence behaviour, this does not mean that nothing can be done about it. A striking example is that of phenylketonuria (or PKU). PKU is a condition caused by inheriting a certain variant of a gene from both parents. Those born with this disorder can accumulate an unusually high level of a substance called phenylalanine in their blood. Phenylalanine is found in foods such as dairy, fish and meat, and those with this disorder are unable to break it down. A build-up of phenylalanine can lead to permanent brain damage resulting in learning disabilities. It's potentially very serious and other symptoms include behavioural difficulties as well as epilepsy. Fortunately most babies are now screened for this at birth via a heel-prick test. Knowledge of this condition allows diets to be changed in order to limit foods containing high levels of phenylalanine and, by doing this, it is possible to avoid the ill effects of this genetic condition. So, PKU may be caused by genes and addressed by environmental means. In the same way, children's sleeplessness may be influenced by the genes that they are born with, yet resolved by behavioural interventions.

From twins we have learned a lot about why sleep differs between children. And it seems that genes are important in helping to explain why some people sleep for longer than others and why some appear to have the gift of good sleep whereas others suffer terribly from disturbed slumber.[13] But, what have twin studies told us about the importance of environmental influences on our sleep? These studies typically highlight that our environment is likely to be even more important than our genes in explaining differences between us in terms of our sleep. Going back to the twin study from researchers at University College London, it was found that twins are alike in terms of their sleep for reasons that are not related to their genes. In other words, aspects of their environment were making twins within a family sleep in a way that was similar to one another.

Which genes? Which environment?

So, we know that both genes and the environment are likely to have an effect on our slumber, but which genes and which aspects of the environment? To start with, which of the approximately 20,000 genes that we are born with are important? This might seem like a simple question, but it's not currently possible to provide robust evidence about many of the genes that are important in explaining the differences between us in terms of sleep quality. To some, that sounds pretty rum and has even been considered a reason to discredit genetic research of this type. One reason for this slow progress is that so many genes are likely to be important and each typically explains only a tiny amount of what is going on.

Scientists have historically searched for genes that are important in explaining differences between us without using the right tools – we've been carving steak with a butter knife. We've focused on just a handful of genes at a time. Instead, we should have been looking at the bigger picture and studying many more of the genetic differences between us, to see if these can explain why our sleep differs. We've also underestimated how many people are required to carry out these studies. It's now clear that huge numbers of volunteers are needed to be able to identify genes involved in complex behaviours. Scientists just didn't know how small the effects were that they needed to be looking for.

To understand genetic influences on sleep quality, scientists might have previously obtained DNA from the

equivalent number of people as those making up two
football teams. If one team (let's call it Snore City) slept well,
whereas another (Insomniacs United) slept poorly, the
scientists might have investigated whether a handful of
genetic variants explained the difference between the two
teams' sleep. They'd ask whether a genetic variant (let's call
it 'slumbertime') was more common in those playing for
Snore City than Insomniacs United. This is referred to as an
association study. It's now known that many of these studies
were carried out on too small a scale and did not provide
enough data for us to be able to detect associations. They
were unable to tell us much about the genetics of sleep
quality, for example. What's more, it was hard to decide
which genetic variants to focus on in these studies. Instead,
we need to collect DNA from many more people than this
(perhaps the tens of thousands of supporters in a stadium) so
that we have more data to work with. We also need to look
at genetic differences across the entire genomes of these
people, rather than focusing on the slumbertime genetic
variant alone.

These newer studies looking at hundreds or thousands of
genetic variants are known as genome-wide association
studies (GWAS) and have provided information about
different aspects of sleep. A GWAS meta-analysis in children
aged 2–14 years old focused on sleep duration and found an
association between a genetic variant on one of the 23 pairs
of chromosomes called chromosome 11 and sleep duration.[14]
However, this was not replicated in two separate samples,
suggesting that perhaps there was no true effect after all, or
that the effects were too small to be detected in the smaller
samples used to attempt replications.

Other GWAS studies have focused on different aspects of
sleep in different age groups. Research led by a team from
Amsterdam examined DNA from more than 100,000 adults
(some suffering from insomnia and some not) in an attempt to
specify genes associated with insomnia.[15] They identified
seven such genes, five of which were supported by looking at
the DNA of a further sample of people.

In addition to increasing the scale of studies, we also need to spend more time considering the endless and sometimes daunting complexities that we now know to exist. Having certain genes may not be a problem for sleep unless we happen to have certain other genes, which when they get together cause trouble. It's like having certain friends with whom we are more likely to get up to mischief!

As well as specifying genes that might be important in sleep, lots of aspects of one's environment have been highlighted as important too. As one example, a consistent bedtime routine might be helpful. This was examined in a study of more than 10,000 mothers of children from birth to five years of age.[16] The mothers, who came from multiple countries, were asked about the activities that took place prior to lights out. They were also asked about the patterns and quality of their offspring's sleep. Children who had a consistent bedtime routine had an earlier bedtime, took less time to fall asleep, woke up less often during the night and slept for longer overall. They also appeared to have fewer problems with their sleep and behaviour during the day. Strikingly, there was a 'dose–response' relationship – this means that the more often a child had a bedtime routine, the better that child slept. Although correlation does not mean causation, one possible interpretation is that a bedtime routine in place once or twice a week might be better than never, but following a routine each night might produce the most soundly sleeping children.

The effects of parenting on children's sleep is not always straightforward and there isn't a universal solution to struggles. Consider a family where the parents put their two children (who we'll call Amy and Bea) to bed at 7 p.m. As a natural lark and long sleeper, Amy might happily fall asleep straight away and wake up feeling refreshed in the morning. The bedtime routine would likely have a positive influence on Amy's sleep quality. Now consider that the other child, Bea, is a natural owl and short sleeper. Bea might argue with her parents before bedtime and spend time thrashing about in bed before succumbing to sleep. This identical bedtime

routine and parenting practice might have a negative influence
on Bea's sleep quality. The same parenting behaviour can
affect people in different ways, as parents who have tried to
sleep-train infants will know, and routines need to be tailored
to the individual.

Important features of the environment can include way
more than the usual suspects of imposing a good routine and
creating a tranquil, dark, quiet and temperate environment.
Even experiences in the womb can be important. With
regards to prenatal experiences, I collaborated on a study
midway through the 2000s where we considered how
experience in the womb might be associated with sleep
problems. The study was led by the scientist Professor Tom
O'Connor from the University of Rochester Medical Center
in New York state. It was based on knowledge from animal
models that indicate stress during pregnancy predicts sleep
patterns in offspring. Seeking to see if similar rules applied to
people, we asked mothers to report whether they'd suffered
from anxiety or depression during their pregnancies. We
then investigated if this was linked to parents' reports of their
babies' sleep once they had been born.[17] In line with what had
been learnt from animals, we found that the mothers who
said they'd been more anxious or depressed during pregnancy
had children who were reported to wake up more during the
night. This was found when the youngsters were both one
and a half and two and a half years old. Interestingly, anxiety
and depression during pregnancy did not seem to be associated
with babies' shut-eye when they were six months old. Perhaps
this was because so many babies of that age have disturbed
sleep, it was impossible to determine significant problems
among other cases. Interestingly we also found that prenatal
anxiety and depression were associated with a general measure
of sleep problems (including difficulties going to sleep,
waking during the night or early in the morning and
nightmares), but not the length of time that a child was
reported to sleep. The research team considered a few
explanations for our results. We looked to see whether they
could be explained by mothers feeling depressed after they'd

had their babies, or because of other issues, such as drinking a lot of alcohol or living in crowded conditions, which might have led to problems. They could not. Instead, in pregnant women, exposure to the 'stress hormone' cortisol, released by the body in response to anxiety and depression perhaps had an effect on the developing foetus, which resulted in disrupted sleep. Such findings underscore the importance of obtaining professional help during pregnancy should mothers experience anxiety or depression.

Nature AND nurture

As we in the field have tried to make sense of genetic and environmental influences, we've found ourselves abandoning the notion of a simplistic nature-versus-nurture all-out war. In its place we've constructed a more nuanced appreciation that both nature and nurture are important, and what's more – they interact. This is to say that genes are not separate from the environment. The genes we are born with may make us more likely to be exposed to certain aspects of the environment (such as being shouted at to go to bed) as well as our sensitivity to that (whether we give a damn about the shouting). Questions, techniques and understanding develop all the time. By the time I retire, the field will be unrecognisable from the one I am involved in today.

When is there really a problem?

We know that infants are likely to differ in terms of their sleep, which can lead to great parental smugness or to desperation. But when does an infant really have a sleep problem that needs to be addressed? Certainly, a large proportion of parents think their child has a sleep problem. Corroborating this, when parents of babies and toddlers were asked if their child had a sleep problem, a big proportion said yes.[3] This ranged from 11 per cent of those asked in Thailand, to a whopping 76 per cent of those asked in China. But defining sleep problems in babies and toddlers is not always simple. Imagine an infant who refuses to fall asleep unless they are being cuddled and who wakes up once during the night wanting a hug. Is that a problem? The answer will depend on whether parents want and expect to engage in this.[18] Some might accept or even like this approach to infant sleep. Ask them if this ritual is a problem and you'll get a resounding 'no!'. Others might hope and expect to put their children in a cot and not see them until the morning. They will find a child's reluctance to settle alone frustrating. Those in the latter camp may find this experience torturous and flag this to friends and paediatricians as a significant problem. Yet the infant has the identical pre-sleep preferences in both scenarios. Different responses to infant sleep are likely to be linked to different approaches to parenting, and perhaps even to life more generally. These discussions result in furious debate. Some parents may be led by instinct, whereas others might want to supplement this with established techniques. It is likely that both groups are making their decision based on what they consider to be in the best interests of their families.

Culture is important here too, and examples of differences include co-sleeping (or sleeping side-by-side or in the same room), which is more common in certain countries than others. For example, in one study of children up to three years old, co-sleeping occurred in fewer than one in ten New Zealanders, but more than eight in ten of those from Vietnam.[3] Bedtime was also found to show cultural variation, with average bedtimes of around 7.30 p.m. for children from New Zealand and around 10.15 p.m. for those from Hong Kong. As reported in *The Atlantic*, even the noise we make when snoring is described differently depending on the culture: *gu gu* in Japanese, *chrrr* in Polish and *de reu rung* in Korean.[19]

Age is important when thinking about sleep too. A baby who sleeps through the night may be a parents' dream, but if that baby is newly born this could be worrying. Certainly, small infants need to wake up: their bellies are tiny and without waking for milk they could become weak and dehydrated. Even older infants and children do not need to sleep for excessively long periods and doing so may at times suggest that there is a problem. Guidelines on how long people of different ages should sleep[1,20] wisely incorporate the idea that one child's need may differ from that of another.

Perhaps there is a reason to move away from thinking of certain aspects of infants' sleep as heroes and villains. There are understandable reasons why infants sometimes refuse to sleep when put down and left to their own devices. Certain theories focus on the need to feel safe in order to sleep, with the common idea that we can 'sleep again' after a threat is no longer present. It certainly is unwise to fall asleep if we don't feel safe. Sleep makes us vulnerable – our vigilance is low and we are unlikely to spy a lion creeping up, the ceiling falling down or, more likely, an attack from a disgruntled older sibling. While infants will not be able to consider the complexities of environmental threats, resistance to being left alone might make good sense in this context. Similarly, the persistence and determination shown by a child who will resolutely refuse to follow a sleep-training schedule may be the same essence that makes that child go on to obtain a gold medal at the Olympics. Moving back to consider genetic research, the same genes that are associated with certain problems can also offer certain advantages. A high genetic loading for anxiety could mean that we are more likely to revise feverishly for exams, and could be useful from an evolutionary perspective, with certain people particularly attentive to, and aware of environmental threats.

So perhaps a waking infant is not a bad thing. It is likely that children will stop waking us during the night at some point. In the same way that parents should be reassured that babies who become mobile and roll over later than others are likely to be able to achieve this skill at some point – why does it matter so much that it happened at three months or five?

However, sleep also needs to be considered in the family context. A child's sleep patterns and sleeplessness may not only affect that child, but also the parents, siblings and possibly even the neighbours too. A parents' health is also important and it's impossible to help a child if we ourselves are not OK. This was brought home to me clearly when talking to 38-year-old Thea, an accountant at a top London firm who decided to pack it in and move to the south of France to become a full-time parent. She did this with gusto and her home not only resembles a scene from a glossy magazine, but has even been featured in one. When each of her three sons was born, she fed them as they fell asleep and they co-slept throughout the night. However, Thea became ill with ulcerative colitis when her youngest son George was just a few months old and she had to leave the family home for urgent surgery. She was devastated at the thought of leaving George and felt that by not rocking and feeding him to sleep she was somehow letting him down. However, by the time she returned from hospital, her husband had managed to put George into what Thea described as a 'perfect routine'. Although a somewhat dramatic example, families sometimes have to play a balancing act, considering the multiple needs and pressures of different members when considering an infant's sleep.

Different techniques can produce positive outcomes and even within a family parents sometimes tailor their approach to bedtime for different children. Feeding and cuddling a child to sleep each night is done with kindness and love, and is a choice for many. Others may consider that letting a child cry for a period can help them learn that they are able to fall asleep without intervention. So if it works best for a family to do what they can to encourage babies to sleep independently through the night, what are the best techniques?

Sleep safe

Before considering the techniques available to help with children's sleep – safety needs to be at the forefront of our minds. Any Brit of my generation will remember with horror the cot death of four-month-old Sebastian, the son of the UK TV presenter Anne Diamond.[21] There is something about a TV presenter that makes us feel that they are part of the family. We share our breakfasts with these people – they are in our bedrooms and living rooms first thing in the morning – and the public sorrow was immense. As reported by the BBC, following this tragedy, a grieving mother found the strength to promote safe sleeping practices in infants. The campaign was called 'Back to Sleep'. It highlighted the importance of laying a baby on its back to sleep. Countless deaths were prevented as a result of this campaign. The statistics speak to that: in the UK, more than 1,500 cases of sudden infant death syndrome (SIDS) were reported to have occurred in 1989,[21] just two years before the death of Sebastian; this had reduced to 214 cases in 2015.[22]

Guidelines about SIDS are constantly reviewed in line with best evidence and so change over time. Recent guidelines include, among other recommendations, making sure that infants are placed on their back for every sleep and letting infants sleep only on firm surfaces – such as appropriate mattresses in cribs that have been safety approved.[23] It's also been suggested that infants should sleep in their own space (such as their own crib), but in the same room as a caregiver. It's important that an infant does not overheat as they sleep, and soft objects such as toys and loose bedding, pillows and bumper pads should be avoided and kept well away from infants during the night.*

In an attempt to help keep babies safe, hospital staff in certain parts of the world are now sending new parents home with a cardboard box.[25] This idea originated in Finland in the 1930s when the government provided parents with a box full of all of the bits and bobs needed for the arrival of their new baby. The boxes had the added benefit of providing a decent location for the babies to sleep too. Sleeping in boxes perhaps conjures up images of the inadvisable practice of allowing babies to sleep in dresser drawers in years gone by. Although schemes similar to that in Finland have since been adopted in Scotland, Argentina and New Jersey, not everyone is happy

---

* Advertisers need to catch up on the importance of promoting safety and stop portraying unsafe sleep environments, such as bumper pads and loose bedding, when marketing infant cribs.[24] Much as it might look cute to show a baby dreaming among a sea of soft toys, this isn't a scenario that should be encouraged in case of accidental suffocation. It simply isn't worth the risk.

with this initiative. Sceptics point out that any apparent
benefits of this scheme may be coincidental and reflect general
improvements in healthcare. Charities have also raised
questions about safety testing and argue that Moses baskets
and cots are the best place for a baby to sleep.[26]

What are the options when getting a child to sleep?

Once safety has been considered, what are the options for
getting a child to sleep? One project I have been involved in,
led by Dr Jodi Mindell, chair of the Paediatric Sleep Council,
provides information at a freely available website (www.
babysleep.com). Here, advice is collated from top paediatric
sleep experts worldwide. Check it out if you are interested in
infant sleep. Physicians, psychologists and researchers have
answered hundreds of questions about sleep via video or text.
You'll find tips about bedtime routines, light and temperature,
transitional objects, night weaning, naps, nappies, books,
dummies, co-sleeping, listening to music at bedtime, and so
much more. Understanding more about such things can be
incredibly useful in helping to create a healthy sleep routine
and this information alone can be enough for parents to feel
they can cope with their baby's sleep.

But what if parents want further advice? There are other
resources, and bookshops are piled high with advice on dealing
with children's weird and wonderful sleep patterns and
problems. But which of these is the best? And what about
when the advice conflicts? To answer such questions, it can be
useful to consider what the science tells us. It's sometimes
argued that we can find a research paper to justify any argument
and that's true to an extent. Couldn't a high-fat diet make us
obese in the 1990s but quite thin in the early 2000s? Because
of this, it's always terrific when scientists spend months of their
lives carefully reading and digesting all the available literature
on a topic and sharing their findings. Over a decade ago, a task
force appointed by the American Academy of Sleep Medicine
did just this and looked at behavioural treatments for problems
at bedtime and wakings during the night in babies and young

children.[27] The aim was to understand how best to manage these issues that are so commonly raised by parents in the clinic. They found strong evidence supporting the effectiveness of behavioural interventions, which were considered useful in reducing resistance at bedtime and wakings during the night in 94 per cent of the studies reviewed.

Two techniques had the greatest empirical support for their aims, although other techniques received support, but to a lesser extent. The first technique to receive the greatest support can be used before a child is even born, to help the family think about the baby's sleep once they arrive. This is **parental education** and involves letting parents know more about their children's sleep and the options available to them to get into good habits and to deal with problems should they occur. For example, if parents are told to put their infant down for the night while they are sleepy but not actually asleep, the infant is more likely to learn from the very start to drift off to sleep without parental involvement. This can be useful not only when putting a baby to bed at night, but also during the night. Sleep cycles mean that people naturally stir during the night. If babies are able to fall asleep alone, they are less likely to need a carer to help them fall back to sleep if they wake up during the night. Learning signs that a child is sleepy doesn't take long. A yawn might be an international sign of tiredness, but signs can also be unique. Whereas one of my sons twiddles his hair, the other rests his right hand on his left collarbone.

The other technique that had the strongest empirical support for its effectiveness was **extinction** or what some refer to as 'crying it out'. This is perhaps the most controversial technique. It involves turning off the lights at night and trying not to react to any sounds that might come from the child's bedroom. That might include singing, giggling and laughing, but more realistically crying. The child may initially cry and shout, but eventually they learn to fall asleep alone. This 'unmodified' version of extinction is not recommended because of the stress it can cause to both parties. Of course, if parents do decide to follow this or similar approaches they shouldn't forget that infants need to be fed during the night in the early months of life, so this approach is not suitable for the very young. In fact, while clinicians may offer advice on how to prevent sleep problems from developing in young infants, they are unlikely to suggest techniques to 'resolve' these problems in very little ones, such as those under six months. Extinction (including the modified version, such as having parents stay in the room) can be effective in bringing about its aims in older infants, but be warned: parents don't always want to use this technique and some find it difficult to implement. Discussing this technique with a parent, I was told: 'I tried this technique out of total desperation – and my daughter cried for ages before falling asleep. Then in the morning I found she was wet from head to toe!' This is a good reminder that if using this technique we should always be aware of a child's needs, checking that they are not ill, stuck in the cot rails, or needing a nappy change.

Other behavioural techniques also received empirical support, although less so than the techniques described previously. One technique that is considered more palatable to some is **graduated extinction**. This is a similar technique, except that parents may keep checking on their children, but with less frequency and less engagement over time. So, even if a child is screaming we initially have to wait for a certain period of time (say five minutes) before we can go and see them. Once we leave them again we'll have to wait for an extended period (say 10 minutes) before we can return. The next time we'll have to wait even longer (say 15 minutes). A colleague followed this technique to the letter, entering the room to check on her children exactly on schedule. She sat outside their rooms wearing earplugs to avoid the stress of hearing her offspring cry. Plotting the data from this experience, she found that they took slightly less time to fall asleep each night (just as we would expect if we were teaching an animal a new skill). After about a week, her children could be put down and would nod off without a fuss.

Positive routines and bedtime fading are also considered useful techniques. The positive routine part of the method aims to create something enjoyable for the child, which hopefully they begin to associate with sleep. Unsurprisingly, the routines often suggested are relaxing – such as having a bath and a peaceful bedtime story. This makes sense, but life comes in all shades. I recall my own routine as a young child wasn't so obviously soporific. My older sister and I would wait eagerly at the top of the stairs until we saw a darkened figure approaching the door. This would trigger a race down the stairs to be the first to cuddle my father upon his return from work. My father, having completed national service earlier in life, would jovially request a military salute before rewarding this obedience with an old army song while lugging one or both of us over his shoulder, up the stairs to bed.

But, family quirks aside, it seems that certain behaviours are popular at bedtime. Certainly stories are often a central component of the bedtime ritual and children often ask to be read the same story again and again. This can get boring for parents, but can offer advantages for children. A study published in 2014 found that repeating a story and allowing sleep soon afterwards helped young children to learn words.[28]

The exact routine employed by a family depends on many factors and will change over time. Slipping into ironed paisley pyjamas at 8 p.m. might be the perfect end to an evening for a schoolboy, but is not so ideal for a man at university trying to secure a partner.

So, whereas there are differences between families, it is clear what the positive routine component of the method involves. But what about the bedtime fading? This involves calling time on bedtime struggles and just putting children to bed when they are tired. The idea is that if we don't let babies compensate for their late bedtime by sleeping on into the morning, they will be tired earlier the next night and go to bed earlier, and so on. A consistent wake time is key and eventually babies will sleep at a time that is acceptable to us.

Another technique involves **scheduled awakenings**. This may sound ridiculous to parents who have spent all evening trying to get their offspring to sleep, as it involves us waking them before we expect them to wake themselves. In other words, if children tend to go to sleep at 7 p.m., but then wake up at 11 p.m., we should wake them up before 11 p.m. and put them back to sleep. Beat them to the punch! The logic is that instead of them waking and making a fuss, we do it for them. We can then settle them back down to sleep without any drama.

More recently, researchers used a statistical technique called a meta-analysis to draw conclusions using data from several studies.[29] This report was led by Dr Lisa Meltzer, paediatric psychologist at National Jewish Health. The team looked at studies addressing insomnia in those from birth to five years of age. It was clear that behavioural techniques helped children to fall asleep more quickly, wake up less often at night and, following awakenings, go back to sleep again more quickly.[29] Perhaps the children had learnt that they did not need their parents to be with them in order to fall asleep when they woke at night. Unfortunately, there were too few studies for the researchers to be able to say which of the behavioural techniques worked best. It was also unclear whether certain methods were particularly good for specific age groups. However, it is quite likely that what works for a new toddler may not work for a child about to begin school. Is it possible consequences of sleep training go beyond the infants and have an effect on the caregivers? A study found that a brief intervention aimed at improving sleep when infants were aged seven months was associated with less depression in mothers when the infants were aged two compared with a control group.[30] However, it has also been flagged that we need much more research to fully understand the long-term family outcomes of different choices for children's sleep.[31]

As to why behavioural approaches work, they all rest on learning principles that focus on the links between a stimulus and a response. They work on the idea of conditioning, where reinforced behaviour is strengthened and ignored behaviour dies out. If we cuddle our screaming children, they learn that if they cry they will be picked up. If we ignore them, they learn that their crying will not lead to a response and so eventually stop. Not everyone is comfortable with this idea though, arguing, for example, that we need to respond to a baby's cries so that they know we are listening, rather than trying to discourage them from communicating in this way. Discussing this with Professor Sarah Blunden, head of paediatric sleep research at CQ University in Australia, she says: 'The interesting thing about sleep training is that we expect a child – particularly a young child – to be able to differentiate the response they get at night (potentially ignoring) with that received in the day (wanting comfort for some other reason, perhaps pain or fear).' Instead of ignoring, it is argued by some that parents should understand that a baby will need around-the-clock care for some time, and that they should perhaps accept this reality rather than try to change a child's sleep schedule in line with their own needs. However, others consider this unfeasible, when up against a short maternity leave, a lack of social support and a busy full-time job.

When considering sleep-training methods, parents sometimes worry that there might be negative consequences. Can their baby cope with the stress? Can they as parents? Will that strong attachment that they are so proud to have formed be obliterated? Acknowledging the significance of these questions for parents, Professor Michael Gradisar, director and clinical psychologist at the Child and Adolescent Sleep Clinic at Flinders University, decided to investigate. He told me: 'Despite claims that sleep training caused attachment problems between parents and their children, there was no direct evidence supporting this. These claims were based on indirect evidence derived from children from deprived or violent living situations, or even animal studies (i.e. rats). We wanted to know what happens when supportive families do sleep training – are there benefits to their sleep, yet costs to their relationships?' In a small study, Gradisar and his team asked parents to put their infants down to sleep using graduated extinction or bedtime fading. There was another group where parents were given sleep education but allowed to put their infants to bed how they liked.[32] The families were then contacted a year later. The sleep training techniques seemed to work best: children in the graduated extinction and bedtime fading groups (but not the education group) drifted off more quickly than they had previously. It was reassuring that when researchers measured the stress hormone cortisol in the infants, they found that those in the sleep technique groups did not seem to have a serious increase over time. The key concern of many parents was whether their attachment with their child would be compromised or whether the children would develop problems with their behaviours and emotions. Both concerns seem to have been unfounded. There were no differences in secure attachment or child problems between the groups when followed up at the age of one. In a further study addressing the long-term implications of infant sleep intervention (provided when infants were seven months old), researchers from Australia assessed families multiple times until the infants were six years of age.[33] Again, there was no indication of negative consequences of behavioural interventions for sleep for either the children or their parents (although of note, long-term benefits to sleep were also not reported as compared with those in the control group).

Discussing these results, Dr Sarah Blunden says: 'Evidence suggests there are no long-term negative effects of sleep training because babies and parents can adapt over time after the immediate effect of the crying has passed ... and that is great and comforting. But the crying at the time itself, is so hard to bear ... that is why efforts to find effective non-ignoring methods that are evidenced-based are important and I'm working on a project investigating exactly that right now.'

In contrast to these reassuring findings, results from a further study caused some concerns. The study involved assessing the stress hormone cortisol in infants and mothers during a five-day sleep-training programme.[34] There was initially synchrony between the cortisol levels of mothers and infants. After a period of sleep training, infants stopped crying when they were put down. However, their cortisol levels did not go down. By contrast, the cortisol levels of the mothers, who no longer witnessed crying infants, decreased, becoming out of line with those of their children.

Not all agree that the results of this study are as problematic as they might first appear. Considering this work, researchers including Gradisar noted a number of issues with the research, such as the use of unmodified extinction (a technique that is not recommended, especially with infants as young as four months old).[35] They also noted that the study did not show that the infants had 'high' levels of cortisol as there is a lack of normative data on this topic. In a game of academic ping-pong, some of the original authors of the work published a response.[36] They agreed that their results did not yet have implications for policy or practice, but noted that their work raised important questions to be further studied. Reviewing the literature as a whole it is clear that further high-quality research is essential in order for parents to make their decisions.

Guts to follow your gut?

While we need to learn more, it seems that sleep training can result in little ones making less fuss at bedtime and being less likely to call out for their parents during the night. Some evidence also suggests that this training is associated with lower levels of maternal depression. Some concerns parents have about using these techniques may also be unfounded. But what about good old gut instinct? Some of what we have learnt to date suggests that if we want to increase our chances of having a child who will visit the land of nod without a song and dance, we should be willing to put them down and leave them to it. And, when sleep training, that sometimes means even if they cry. However, speak to the majority of parents and they will find this uncomfortable and in some cases agonising. They might refer to an intuition that this doesn't feel right. So should we really ignore this instinct when it comes to sleep? To do so flies in the face of so much else that is taught about child rearing. Take a baby to the doctor when they are small and you might be told that 'you should follow your gut instinct'. We are so often encouraged and praised for following our intuition. As to what this is, perhaps it is a reaction to evidence and something that has developed to help us survive. It is certainly useful in some cases.

Gut instinct can be wrong too of course. One parent recalled how she had followed the sage advice received from her doctor and 'followed her gut', and was bright pink with embarrassment to admit she had called the emergency services following the first time her son had a bottle of milk and choked rather dramatically on it. He was of course fine. And how many of us would have missed out on our jobs if we'd followed our intuition and stayed at home instead of going to an interview? So perhaps 'gut instinct' is sometimes an emotional response rather than a balanced consideration of the evidence and should not always be followed blindly. We should be both thinking with our head and reacting to what our gut tells us in order to navigate the early parenting years.

Sleep easy

Dealing with sleep in infancy is not easy. Parents who have engaged in the modified extinction technique can be horrified that a holiday or a minor illness can entirely throw their schedule. Some worry that ignoring their children's cries at night could teach their offspring that their needs will not be met and consequently disadvantage them later in life. And what about different folks, different strokes? It may suit one family to extinguish their child's sleeplessness with a carefully hatched plan, but not others. One of my sons experienced occasional seizures during the night when he was small (something that has ceased over time) and that left me with an unhealthy neuroticism about his sleep. Nobody would advocate risking the safety of children by leaving alone those who need us by their side. However, once they are considered to be well and not at risk, those following sleep-training schedules are sometimes advised to let their child cry for a while so that they can learn to sleep without parental intervention. But this is not always easy.

Many struggle to sleep-train their children, but what about those who don't want to train their children? Perhaps they don't mind, or even enjoy cuddling their children while they fall asleep – as was the case for Thea the ex-accountant. Should these parents worry about giving their children a disadvantage in life by not encouraging them to fall asleep alone? Will this set them up for a life of sleeplessness? Are our behaviour patterns really established when we are young so that the child is 'father of the man' when it comes to our sleep? Instead, parents might be comforted by the suggestion that sleep can be changed over time. They may want to provide assistance when an infant is young or sick or on holiday, but that does not mean that they can't decide on a different approach later in their child's development. Studies are only just beginning to systematically address questions that are so fundamental in helping parents to make their choices and there remain as many unanswered questions as answered ones.

Thinking back to my appointment with the sonographer many moons ago, the reference to sleep now makes more sense. I had been all too aware of the scientific literature on sleep before that meeting, but I was clueless about the reality of dealing with a sleepless baby. Other parents were consumed by this topic and lamenting their own sleep loss too. There are important reasons why a baby wakes up during the night and many reasons to celebrate this occurrence. There are reasons why one child sleeps in a different way to another, and caregivers are unlikely to have done anything 'wrong' to bring this about. That is not to say that an infant's sleeping pattern can't be altered and, after considering safety, what is right for one family may differ from what is right for another. Our uniqueness is surely a reason to celebrate.

CHAPTER THREE

Preschool and School-Aged Children: The Rainbow of Sleep Problems

Preschool children (3–5 years) recommended 10–13 hours of sleep per 24 hours
School-aged children (6–12 years) recommended 9–12 hours of sleep per 24 hours [1]

How do preschool and school-aged children sleep?

'Will you lie next to me, Daddy?'
'I've had a nightmare and I'm scared of the dark.'
'There was a great big bang in my head when I was falling asleep.'
'I've seen a ghost and I don't want to sleep by myself.'

The challenges of a waking baby can be replaced by a rich array of other sleep problems. Sleep changes immensely during the period between infancy and the teenage years, and a lot can go wrong – from restless legs to exploding heads. So what have we learned about this period of life and is there really a scientific explanation for having seen that ghost?

As children grow they spend progressively less time asleep. The 11–14 hours per day recommended for one- to two-year-olds[1] decreases to 10–13 hours by the age of three to five years old. This leaves parents with one fewer hour to enjoy eating their own dinner, or wiping their child's dinner off the kitchen walls. Children will stop napping too, and whereas one-year-olds typically have a morning and afternoon nap, one of these is usually dropped around the time that the 'terrible twos' are kicking off. By three to six years of age, naps are usually a thing of the past. As infants grow, they are

also likely to move on from their cots and be footloose in a
bed – this often occurs around the age of three or four.

By the time children are heading off for their first day at
school, things may be looking up for parents. The children
are at school during the day, providing their carers new-found
time to take control of their home or return to that elusive
career. With a bit of luck, a school-aged child will have been
sleeping through the night without interruption for some
time too. Reaching this significant sleep milestone is often a
parenting highlight.

Of course, how sleep patterns develop depends, in part,
on where we happen to have grown up. Long daytime naps,
for example, may suit some people living in Spain. A daytime
sleep is common around the world and may have many
benefits, from helping to improve our mood, to increasing
alertness and performance. However, the late bedtimes that
sometimes accompany the siesta may horrify certain parents
living in the UK. It's not that one is right and the other is
wrong. Instead, perhaps these long-established habits can be
difficult to shake, or these patterns may be more appropriate
in some circumstances than others. I recently spoke to
Emilio, a father of two who lives in Spain and holidays in
the UK for a month each year. His take on the siesta was
that it makes good sense in Spain but perhaps not in England.
He told me: 'It can get really hot in Spain. Who wants to
be out in 40-degree heat during the day? It's better to be
asleep.' He continued: 'But, equally, who wants the kids
wide awake at 9 p.m. in the UK? Everything is shut! There
is nothing for them to do. Tire them out during the daytime
instead.'

During early childhood, sleep also changes in ways that we
can't see and the trend of decreasing REM sleep continues. It
also takes progressively longer to move through the 'sleep
cycle' (which involves cycling through REM and NREM
stages of sleep). Whereas a premature baby might complete a
sleep cycle halfway through a football match (it takes some of
them around 45 minutes), we'll have to wait for the final
whistle for adolescents to complete theirs (at approximately

90 minutes). It stays that way for the rest of life. This means that when thinking about sleep we need to remember that babies and children are not just mini-adults.

What sleep problems might children experience?

Of course, much can go wrong with sleep. Any clinician working with patients with sleep disorders is likely to be familiar with *The International Classification of Sleep Disorders,* which is currently in its third edition.[2] This contains more sleep disorders than most people would have thought existed. These disorders are categorised into a number of major categories, specifically insomnia, sleep-related breathing disorders, central disorders of hypersomnolence (involving daytime sleepiness), circadian-rhythm sleep–wake disorders, parasomnias (characterised by unwanted physical experiences and events occurring during or in the transition into and out of sleep), sleep-related movement disorders and other sleep disorders. The disorders listed range from those that most people have certainly heard of and possibly even experienced, such as insomnia, to those that they almost certainly won't. (More on 'exploding head syndrome' later.) Although different sleep disorders can occur in people of different ages, they are discussed in this chapter because some of these problems can first appear early in life.

Can't sleep, won't sleep: sleep refusal and insomnia

When we think about insomnia we might conjure up an image of a chronically stressed adult lying in bed tossing and turning. Insomnia presents problems in getting to sleep, staying asleep or waking up too early. However, things can be quite different with children. When we look at classification systems used to define insomnia in children, they include descriptions of declining to sleep at an appropriate time or refusing to sleep alone. These are common symptoms, which perhaps help to explain why the parody book *Go the F*** to Sleep*[3] was such a runaway success among parents.

So, if children won't comply with a 7 p.m. bedtime, or they beg a parent to lie next to them as they fall asleep, are they showing symptoms of insomnia? Of course, those symptoms alone don't constitute insomnia. If they did, every parent in the land would be off seeking help regarding their children's sleep. We could be lulled to sleep right now by going through the diagnostic criteria at length (e.g. symptoms must occur at least three times a week for three months). Researchers are inconsistent when defining insomnia or sleeplessness in their studies, which is one reason why when we look at prevalence rates of insomnia in children they can vary wildly. As with all disorders, how often the problem occurs and how serious it is needs to be considered. Clinicians start to sit up and take notice when the sleep disturbance is having a negative effect on a family's life. This can involve children behaving badly. Perhaps strangely, at least to us adults who when tired so often flop in front of the TV, sleep-deprived children will often seem to be full of beans and appear as if they are 'bouncing off the walls'. This can lead to the worrying conclusion that they are not tired at all and should perhaps be allowed to stay up a little longer.

Not only do sleep problems appear to be linked to a whole host of other problems (discussed later in the book), but some types of insomnia involve children waking up when everyone else is asleep, which can be unsettling for parents. This may simply result in a child nestling happily in between exhausted parents who then miss out on the sleep quality they deserve (and end up lamenting their purchase of a king- rather than super-king-sized bed). However, if a child wakes up but decides on a different course of action, such as playing unsupervised, the consequences of night waking can be more concerning.

So why is it more difficult for some children to go to sleep (and stay asleep) than others? As discussed previously, genes and environmental influences are likely to be important in explaining differences between children. We've considered ways in which aspects of the environment could affect a child's sleep, but the focus has been on things that happen at home. As children grow they typically spend more time away from the family and experiences outside the home can start to influence sleep too. These experiences can make siblings less similar in terms of their sleeping patterns. Research shows that children who are victimised by their peers are likely to sleep less well than those who are not.[4] There could be various reasons for this, but those who are bullied may be more likely than others to worry and ruminate at bedtime. Lying in bed reliving instances of fear, frustration and anger will never aid restful sleep.

Events linked to poor sleep quality are not always stressful – such as bullying – and can include too little time spent playing sport, or lack of exposure to sunlight. But they do, of course, also include those that are severe, and there is a literature, which makes for distressing reading, showing that children who have suffered trauma, whether experiencing war-related stress, a natural disaster or abuse, can struggle to sleep well, both in the short term and also later in life.[5,6]

So, it is pretty clear that both genes and environment are important in explaining differences between people, but why? How does our environment 'get under our skin' and lead to sleep problems? Well, for one, it can affect the way that we think, which can influence the way that we sleep. We know a lot about how this works in adults. Sometimes we 'catastrophise' about not being able to sleep, which is not very conducive to nodding off.[7] Catastrophising involves a 'what if?' thought process. We may lie in bed worrying about what tomorrow is going to be like if we get no sleep. Perhaps we'll feel tired, which might lead to underperforming at work, which may lead to being sacked, financial problems at home, losing the house, losing custody of the children, stress, ill health and so on. We may also think that when we can't sleep we should stay in bed and try harder. This is dysfunctional – as good sleep should be automatic rather than effortful. Good sleepers don't have to try hard to achieve a restful night, they just automatically get one.

By contrast, childhood insomnia is more of an enigma. A while ago it struck me that children with insomnia have been thought of as if they are rats in mazes: parents do one thing that produces exhibit A (a bad sleeper), or another that results in exhibit B (a good sleeper). But little consideration was being given to the thoughts children were having about sleep. One of my first research projects at Goldsmiths, University of London, was therefore to try to understand more about what children were thinking about sleep. Together with a dedicated team of hard-working young students and researchers, I travelled to a few inner-city London schools and asked the children lots of questions about their sleep as well as their bedtime thoughts and beliefs about sleep. We focused on schoolchildren as young as eight years old – any younger and we thought they might not understand our questions. We were fascinated to find that some of what we know about thoughts in adults with insomnia may be relevant to children too. We found that children with poorer sleep also held more dysfunctional beliefs about sleep, just like adults.[8] We found many other interesting parallels too – such as that the children who slept least well tended to catastrophise about their sleep.[9] This seemed to be related to their feelings of anxiety and depression. It was intriguing to learn more about what children think about, and one little girl talked us through her thought processes following not being able to nod off. She thought her sleeplessness would give her a headache and she would not do very well at school the next day. She was worried that this would get her into trouble with her parents, who would then refuse to buy her treats. A more surprising response came from a little boy who was worried that sleeplessness would turn him into the Boogeyman wrestler who eats worms! We also found that the children who slept least well told us they often had thoughts racing through their heads when they were in bed – again, just like adults.[10]

So what should we do with this information? It seems that helping children to unwind before bedtime might be a good start. Bedtime stories are often far from soporific and are pumped up with ideas that probably excite children in the same way that an interesting email arriving just before bedtime does for an adult. Are stories about flying through space, meeting a monster, talking to animals or having a day out at an adventure park really relaxing? And then parents are sometimes surprised or annoyed that their children don't then fall asleep.

But that's just not how sleep works. Children, just like adults, need to take some time to unwind before hitting the hay. This was smartly pointed out by the Swedish author Carl-Johan Forssén Ehrlin[11] who wrote a bestselling book called *The Rabbit Who Wants to Fall Asleep*, designed to help children relax and fall asleep. The book includes characters such as 'Uncle Yawn' and the 'Heavy-Eyed Owl' and the person reading the bedtime story to a child is encouraged to read certain sections slowly and in a calm voice, and to yawn a lot while reading. Developing upon the general idea that children need to unwind before bed, I have co-written an anthology of bedtime stories called *The Sleepy Pebble and Other Stories*, which incorporates techniques aimed at helping children relax at night. During the development stage, the ideas and stories were discussed with other paediatric sleep experts, as well as psychologists, parents of small children and some children themselves. Next, we were interested to see how these stories were received by families and whether they were reported to be useful. We invited 100 families to read one of the stories to their children (between 3 and 11 years of age) for three consecutive nights. At the end of those nights, we asked them to complete a survey including lots of questions, such as what they thought about the length of the stories and how best they should be illustrated. Seventy of those recruited to take part in the study responded. One of our key questions was: 'Overall, what effect do you think the story had on your child/children's sleep?' The parents responded that for 80 of their 104 children (77 per cent) the story had a 'very positive' or 'slightly positive' effect.*

---

* Parents also reported that for 21/104 (20 per cent) the book seemed to have no effect; for 3/104 (3 per cent) the book seemed to have a slightly negative/extremely negative effect/did not comment. These responses are promising, but this was a preliminary report designed to further improve the book and there were limitations (no control group, the use of subjective retrospective reports and recruitment via social media, meaning that the authors were known to some participants).

Around the same time as I was running my study on children's thinking in relation to their sleep, in London, a totally independent team of scientists were researching similar questions. The team was led by psychologist Dr Candice Alfano, who was unknown to me at the time. Alfano is a professor of psychology in Houston. She looked at the associations between sleep and pre-sleep arousal (or feeling wound up before bedtime) in a sample of children suffering from anxiety. She found that poorer sleep was linked to greater mental arousal – especially for children with an anxious personality.[12] Our independent studies in different populations had reached similar conclusions. Our preliminary studies in this area suggest to me that the way children are thinking is important for their sleep. While I stick to my earlier claim that children shouldn't be thought of as mini-adults, perhaps there are more similarities than are sometimes acknowledged: children's thoughts matter too.

When discussing children's refusal to go to sleep when they are told, parents sometimes smirk and roll their eyes. Isn't it just the case that most children dislike sleep? A fair point. Perhaps children think, as indeed some adults do, that it is a royal waste of time that interferes with the important things in life. Surely sleep can't compete with the joys of racing snails, playing superheroes or roly-polying down a hill? In order to know more about children's underlying, implicit, attitudes to sleep I collaborated with Dr Megan Crawford, who is now a lecturer at Swansea University. She developed an ingenious experiment using the implicit-association test. This technique looks at the time people take to categorise various stimuli, which can be used to discover what they really think. This test is often used to look at attitudes that some people may hold but are perhaps not keen to admit, such as those concerning racial or gender biases. The essence of this task is that it takes longer to categorise something in a way that is against our true beliefs than in a way that is consistent with what we believe. So, if we truly believe that sleep equals all things bad, it would take longer to pair a picture of pyjamas with a positive word such as 'good' or 'fun' than with a negative word such as 'yucky' or 'bad'. Using this approach, Crawford found that children were quicker to pair sleep-related pictures (such as an image of a pillow) with bad words than with good words.*

So, it seems that children aren't just telling us they don't like sleep – they might really mean it. This can be difficult to comprehend, as some adults like nothing more than engulfing themselves in the crisp sheets of their beds after a long day. However, the preferences of others can be surprising.[†] To avoid reinforcing the idea that sleep (or perhaps even just the bedroom) is bad, it makes sense that we should do all we can to weaken that link. For example, we should never tell a child that if they misbehave they must 'go to their bedroom', 'go to their cot', or 'go to bed without supper'. After all, sleep is a great pleasure, right? Yes, for some, but sadly I'm not convinced that an early bedtime is likely to become a treat for good behaviour in children any time soon.

A parent's desire for their offspring to go to bed combined with a child's dislike of sleep can make for an explosive bedtime. Some of the behavioural techniques discussed previously, such as bedtime fading, can be helpful when faced with a child refusing to go to bed or to sleep alone. When children are slightly older, significant insomnia may warrant cognitive behaviour therapy – a talking therapy that addresses thoughts and behaviours. This typically involves both parents and children, and comprises a number of components. There

---

* This work is unpublished. Whether this finding will replicate remains to be seen – especially in light of some general criticism levelled towards the use of this test, such as that scores could reflect societal rather than personal views.[13]

† I was recently stunned by my husband's declaration that he would happily replace all food with nutritionally balanced pills.

can be information about sleep hygiene, or rather the practices that optimise the chance of good sleep – such as exposure to light in the day and avoiding it at night. Relaxation techniques, such as breathing exercises, can be taught. Then there is sleep restriction, or the idea that delaying bedtime might be useful if children are not able to sleep on their current schedule. Stimulus control therapy aims to ensure that children only use their bedroom to sleep so that they do not associate it with arousal. Finally, cognitive therapy can help to manage parents' expectations about what they should expect from their children's sleep. This type of technique has been found to be useful in improving sleep behaviour in both the short and long term in children between five and ten years of age.[14]

To increase the chances of good sleep, it's useful to be consistent and firm and do what we can to create an environment that is conducive to getting sound sleep. For a start, it might make sense to avoid TV in bedrooms as there is research showing that preschoolers with a TV in their room were reported to have poorer sleep quality than those without.[15] Going back to the idea that we need to create an environment that makes children feel safe is important too, because if we don't feel safe, it doesn't make sense to lose vigilance by falling asleep. Gru in the film *Despicable Me* is loveable, but his parenting practice of getting the children to sleep in hollowed-out bombs might not quite live up to that recommendation.

One little trick that can be used to help children become sleepy before bed is to dim the lights. The science behind this approach is that bright light can suppress melatonin production, so dimming the lights can allow melatonin to flow joyfully and let the body know it's time to fall asleep.

The good old entrepreneurs have capitalised on the links between light and melatonin and we don't have to look far to see products embracing this knowledge. For example, there are glow-in-the-dark stickers, which marketers profess will result in less melatonin suppression than nightlights; motion activated lights that illuminate the toilet bowl and can be set to produce a soft red glow; as well as many other products. While dimming the lights in a home can help with sleep too, this ritual does pose risks, such as accidentally brushing our teeth with athlete's foot cream or developing signs of eye strain from reading in poorly lit rooms.

So there are things that we can do in the home to increase the chances of our young children falling asleep, but as a society should we be doing more? Campaigns in playgroups, nurseries and schools designed to convince children about the importance of sleep might be a good place to start. Perhaps parents could tell their children that prioritising getting their head down might help them run faster, have more fun with their friends and learn more. But will these techniques work? This is not yet clear. Research suggests that education delivered in school about sleep increases knowledge, but doesn't necessarily translate into improved sleep or reduced problems in associated areas.[16] In other words, children might know that they should go to sleep, but still refuse to do so.

Discussing this with Professor Sarah Blunden, whom I mentioned in Chapter 2, she says: 'The question is why are they not changing their sleep behaviour? The answer might well be that they don't want to give up on things that they perceive to be better than sleep, such as screen time, peer and family interaction. The key in encouraging them to change their behaviour is to be a team: work with them rather than tell them what to do. Give them choices and options and help them choose better sleep behaviour. Children, just like adults, don't want to be told what to do, even if they know it is good for them. But they do want to do the right thing and know that doing so gains our approval. I always say to the children I work with: "Are you tired? Do you like feeling that way? Are you happy with your performance and how you feel? If not, then you have the power to change that. And I have the information to help you." That is a powerful combination for sleep behaviour change.'

Things that go bump in the night: dreams and nightmares

People love talking about their dreams, whether they are about housework, having a bear for a pet, flying across open water or an enduring friendship with Prince Harry. Often the person talking about their dream draws some meaning from the content, or considers it an omen for the future. Certainly, it has been claimed that Abraham Lincoln believed dreams to be extraordinary – something which is particularly poignant as he dreamt that he had been assassinated days before it indeed happened.[17]

Others might claim 'paranormal experiences' wherein, for example, they dreamed of a friend, and soon after found out that friend was pregnant. ('You can't mess with my third eye,' my friend Michelle tells me over afternoon tea, talking about those who like to conceal their pregnancies in the early days, 'my dreams always tell me what is going on.') Not everyone is convinced by the greater meaning of dreams. Scientists are trained to question such 'evidence' and consider the number of people dreamt about who are not pregnant.

A colleague at Goldsmiths, professor of psychology Chris French, whose work focuses on understanding the psychology behind paranormal beliefs and experiences, has explained his stance on this to me. Referring to analyses by US mathematician John Allen Paulos, French points out that someone might be impressed if they had a dream that resembled something that then happened shortly afterwards in their waking life. This might especially be the case if the chance of this happening, and of them remembering this on any given night, were only, let's say, 1 in 10,000. This sounds incredibly unlikely, so when it does occur, people sometimes take this as evidence for the paranormal. However, when we do the maths, working out how this probability pans out over time, we end up with roughly equal odds of having a dream of this type in a 19-year period. That means that if we ask an undergraduate class whether they've had a precognitive dream of this type, a large proportion might say they have. These dreams are rare, but they do occur. A failure to calculate probabilities can help to explain why people may uncritically accept paranormal beliefs.

Even those who are unconvinced by the greater meaning of dreams may be interested in knowing that dreams can tell us about emotional or cognitive development. For example, a study led by scientists from Hungary looked at dreams reported by children aged four to eight years old in relation to their cognitive skills. The types of dreams reported changed with development and reporting one's active self in a dream was a sign of better skills.[18] Dreams also have an interesting association with different aspects of mental health – most notably post-traumatic stress disorder, where dreams of a traumatic event might reoccur time and time again.

And what about nightmares? These are pretty common in pre-adolescent children and are a source of distress. They can disturb sleep for an entire family, with children waking upset and seeking comfort from others. As to what causes nightmares, genes and the environment are of course important, but which aspects? Stressful life events, such as starting at a new nursery or school, or experiencing changes in family circumstances can be important. Not only that, but thinking hard about what a child is exposed to on a day-to-day basis, and perhaps particularly just before they go to bed, may help. Are dramatic TV shows (including watching the Boogeyman wrestler!), playing video games late at night or even reading frightening books likely to help a child sleep well? In fact, anything that can increase anxiety in a child could potentially be problematic, and links have been reported between child anxiety and nightmares.[19] But it is likely that this cuts both ways, with children who experience nightmares also likely to feel more anxious than others.

Talking about sleep can provide a good way for healthcare providers to build a rapport with families. Most people seem happy to talk about this topic, allowing the conversation to get comfortable before moving on to topics that may be more sensitive, such as depression. 'How is your sleep?' is surely a much better way to start an assessment than, 'Are you feeling sad, empty or hopeless?' Perhaps talking about dreams and nightmares might also be a useful way for parents to understand more about what is stressing and upsetting their children. Hearing of repeat nightmares about the big dog next door, a seemingly angelic playmate, or Uncle Leo flying away forever, might help to initiate important discussions.

Parents understanding children's underlying stresses could translate into helping them deal with the things they struggle with. It's good to open this dialogue as some of these stresses may seem alien to adults. A Valentine's card from an admiring friend may produce happy tears from a grown man, but livid ones from a seven-year-old boy.

Typically, nightmares don't need to be treated, except with comfort and reassurance, often in the form of a bear hug, or at least some kind words. However, for serious cases there is help at hand. *A Clinical Guide to Pediatric Sleep*[20] is often regarded as *the* book for experts who deal with children's sleeping issues. This suggests the use of relaxation techniques such as progressive muscle relaxation, which involves tensing and releasing muscles throughout the body to raise awareness of the sensations associated with each state. Imagery rehearsal may also be useful. This involves children playing out frequent nightmares in a more positive way. For example, when they wake from a nightmare, they could replay it and make it more positive, be in greater control or improve the content. This type of psychological treatment has been found to be effective in reducing the frequency of nightmares.[21] My own nightmare of my father dying has been rescripted to remember childhood camping trips, with my impossibly handsome, healthy and happy 40-something-year-old father living in that state for an eternity.

A fright in the night: sleep terrors

Dreams and nightmares mainly occur during REM sleep, the sleep stage where we're paralysed and therefore prevented from acting out our dreams. Sleep terrors are sometimes mistaken for bad dreams, but in fact they are something quite different. We are not paralysed during sleep terrors. In fact, it is exactly for this reason that they may be so alarming to others. The person experiencing these terrors may leap out of bed, shout, scream and look terrified. What's happening is that while someone has been aroused from the deepest stages of NREM, they are not fully awake. These sleep disorders are most likely to occur soon after we go to bed. Their timing makes perfect sense given the composition of our sleep cycles throughout the night. During the beginning of the night we spend much of our time in deep NREM, whereas we spend a larger proportion in REM towards the end of the night.

There are other disorders in this family of diagnoses (known as NREM-related parasomnias). They range from 'confusion arousals', which are pretty similar to sleep terrors except that the sufferer seems confused and groggy rather than fearful, to sleepwalking and even sleep-related eating disorder. Key features of these disorders include that it is difficult to wake someone from an episode. These experiences are also characterised by low-complexity behaviours, which are somewhat automatic, rather than having been carefully planned.

Those observing sleep terrors are often desperate for a solution. Whereas those experiencing terrors will likely wake up in the morning blissfully unaware of the drama of the night, witnessing these events can be distressing. Knowing what triggers sleep terrors, such as poor or disrupted sleep during previous nights or experiencing stress, provides a possible way to prevent them by trying to minimise these triggers. To prevent terrors it can be useful to monitor when they occur and to disrupt sleep before that time. Regardless of how sleep terrors are dealt with, perhaps the best news of all is that we know sleep changes from cradle to grave and that, as we approach adulthood, NREM decreases dramatically, along with the chances of experiencing related sleep disorders.

Walking by night: sleepwalking

If sleep terrors are Tweedledum, sleepwalking is Tweedledee. They are alike in that they both involve arousal during slumber and stem from NREM. Someone sleepwalking might shoot out of bed, or move about in a more leisurely manner. Behaviours can be agitated, aggressive or at times quite relaxed. Actions can be simple or appear complex – and they are often quite bizarre, such as urinating in a dustbin. The person experiencing an episode might end up back in bed, fast asleep and none the wiser – or can wake up somewhere quite unexpected.

Sleepwalking can first occur very early in life. As soon as we can walk, we are potentially able to sleepwalk. In fact, even before that time, some children will sleep-crawl!

It seems that rather than waking up fully from NREM sleep, the sleepwalker is only partially awake. Certain regions of the brain involved in movement are 'awake', whereas others, such as those involved in memory, are not.[22] As with sleep terrors, these events tend to occur in the early stages of a night's sleep when NREM sleep is most abundant. Sleepwalking is common, with up to 40 per cent of children aged 6–16 years old having experienced this disturbance at least once. Regular walkabouts are far less likely (affecting around just 2–3 per cent[23]). While relatively common, sleepwalking is a concern. We have the power to move but without the use of our higher brain functions to keep us safe. Huan, a journalist based in New York, described to me her daughter Lin's sleepwalking, which she only seems to do when tired. Huan tells me that of all her experiences she remembers being most alarmed during a trip to Naples. 'We had a scary event in which Lin walked to the door of the hotel room and started opening it. Luckily my husband woke up and was able to stop her. It was our first night in Italy so she was probably pretty sleep deprived from the overnight flight. We blocked the door the next night, but it was pretty freaky.' Sleepwalking children may choose to avoid fun events such as sleepovers. But talking to a clinician, I hear more concerning stories of adults, such as that of a salesman who drove to his childhood home – the whole time fast asleep. He tells me another case of a man who ended up in his neighbour's apartment in the middle of the night (the police were called), and a final tale of a man who woke up on the roof of his house having made the ascent while sleepwalking.

Despite parents' requests, doctors can be slow to refer patients for assessment in sleep laboratories. This is partly because it is often difficult to tell much from these assessments. For example, on the nights that patients spend in the sleep lab and actually want to sleepwalk, they often do not, something known as 'Sod's Law' in the UK and 'Murphy's Law' in the USA. Instead, it might be worth setting up video recordings in the home and keeping diaries of sleepwalking.

The causes of sleepwalking are similar to those of sleep terrors. They include being stressed or sleep deprived, but they can also be linked to other sleep disorders, such as those involving difficulty breathing at night, or physical problems, perhaps caused by a head injury. It has also been proposed that external stimuli, such as a mobile phone pinging during the night, can disturb sleep and result in arousals. This is just one of many reasons why we should follow the example of the smooth-skinned celebrities such as Daniel Craig and Rachel Weisz and banish technology from the bedroom.[24]

To deal with sleepwalking it can be useful to ensure that sleep practices are as good as they can be.[22] Perhaps the most important thing is to keep the environment safe by bolting the front door, putting child locks on windows and installing stair gates.[20] Alarms can also help by waking up parents who can then calmly encourage their children back to bed without waking them. Drugs may be prescribed in severe cases and nightly cases can be dealt with by waking a child before we think the event is likely to occur. Perhaps most reassuringly, sleepwalking – and sleep terrors – tend to resolve by adolescence or adulthood.

Snoring babies! Sleep-disordered breathing

Sleep-disordered breathing can also occur from the very earliest stages of life. Apnoea, where breathing stops for an alarming number of seconds, is particularly common in premature babies, whose brains may have underdeveloped respiratory centres. Newborn babies' cute little snuffles and snorts can be quite endearing. However, in some cases this can reflect more than having developed a common cold. The physiology of certain babies can make them susceptible to breathing difficulties during sleep. Childhood is the time that adenoids and tonsils are most likely to be enlarged, so this is often a problem during this stage of life. Other reasons for sleep-disordered breathing include a stuffy nose, which could be caused by allergies or a smoke-filled home; facial abnormalities, which can be due to a plethora of disorders, such as Down's syndrome; and obesity, which has increased over the years and might help to explain the rise in sleep-disordered breathing too.

Worrying links have been flagged between sleep-disordered breathing and problematic behaviour.[25] It is possible that children suffering from sleep-disordered breathing experience later difficulties because they are being repeatedly woken up at night and so are not getting the kip they need. Another possibility is that the abnormalities in gas exchange might be playing a role. Sleep-disordered breathing is also linked to other problems, such as neurocognitive difficulties and atypical development of the jawbone. Because of that, when it occurs, doctors should always be made aware of it and should take it seriously. Action should depend on the cause of the problem and how bad it is. One possibility is that a doctor will tell us to wait to see if this is something that a child will grow out of. After all, children's adenoids are heading to that tranquil state of nothingness by the time they become adults, so can no longer bother them. In mild cases, a patient might be given Montelukast and nasal steroids. In certain cases surgery is recommended or the patient may be told to try to lose some weight, as that may be a cause of the problem to begin with.

The still of night

Night-time is often associated with stillness, but for some it's quite the opposite. Some people spend their night running as if in a race, grinding their teeth to stubs or head-banging as if at a concert.

Restless legs syndrome involves an irresistible compulsion to move the legs. Talk to people suffering from this disorder, and they might describe particular problems when sitting or lying down, especially at night. They are also likely to describe a deeply uncomfortable feeling, if the drive to move is not fulfilled. Despite the name, the action is not all in the legs and some people report a similar urge to move the arms or torso too. This disorder is more likely to occur in females than males, is common in pregnant women and is most common among the older population – with links reported to diseases such as Parkinson's, rheumatoid arthritis and multiple sclerosis.[2] When restless legs syndrome occurs in children it is sometimes mistaken for 'growing pains' or symptoms of attention deficit hyperactivity disorder (ADHD).

Vigorous teeth grinding is a common action during the night. This can result in damage to the teeth, a jaw ache and a headache too. Grinding is often linked to stress. Interestingly, it's sometimes also said that people who are highly motivated, the go-getters of the world, also have a vulnerability to this.[2] Sufferers are sometimes recommended relaxation methods as well as other tips; however, evidence supporting the effectiveness of such techniques is mixed.[26]

Head-banging and rocking involves rhythmic movements at night. This often occurs as a baby is trying to get to sleep. It can be alarming to those witnessing the event, with little ones banging their heads into pillows, mattresses, cot bars or even walls. But it is common, and may simply reflect their attempts to soothe themselves to sleep. Such movements can be particularly pronounced in those who have experienced a tough start to life, for example, missing out on a strong and positive relationship with parents, or being raised under circumstances in which they may have experienced high levels of boredom or stress.

At the very beginning of my PhD I worked on a study called the English and Romanian Adoptee Project. This is a study of adopted children living in the UK. Following the fall of communism in Romania, many children ended up in institutions. Televised scenes of their deprivation led to adoptions by families throughout the UK. While involved in the project, I travelled around the UK getting to meet many inspiring families involved in the study. Without exception, I was offered a warm welcome into their homes.

An early report from this study focused on behaviours that have been associated with being raised in an institution. Among findings, parents retrospectively reported that 67 of the 144 children from Romanian institutions rocked their bodies when they entered the UK.[27] This occurred during the day or – of relevance here – at night. Some of the children had not spent very long in the institutions and were adopted at just a few weeks old. Others had been there for a long time and came to the UK when they were older than three years of age.

The longer a child had experienced deprivation, the more likely their adoptive parents were to report that they rocked their bodies. When the researchers looked at two comparison groups they saw a different story. In a group of children adopted from Romania, but who had not spent time in institutional care, only two out of 21 children rocked their bodies. Furthermore, none of the children from a comparison group, adopted within the UK, who had not experienced institutional care, rocked their bodies in this way. This study might tell us more about why this rocking develops and the functions it might serve under certain circumstances.

Waking wet: bedwetting

Another problem that is rife in pre-teens is bedwetting.[28] Most parents will have had the dubious honour of trading deep sleep for dealing with soggy bed linen. Bedwetting is a normal part of childhood and should be handled as such. Making sure that children make that final trip to the toilet before bed and wear nappies if needed are ways to deal with the issue. A midnight tinkle in bed is only really considered a problem when it happens frequently, when we would no longer expect it. The arbitrary cut-off is five years of age – and if a child is regularly bedwetting after that point, talk to a doctor.

Persistent bedwetting is more likely to occur in boys and those who have family members who had the same experience.[29] So if your child is wetting the bed, perhaps you or your partner did too? One explanation for this common problem is an issue with the rate at which someone is maturing, as they may have a relatively small bladder for their age. The bladder could also be compressed for another reason, such as constipation. Those who wet the bed may also be particularly difficult to wake, which might be because of another problem. Sleep-disordered breathing, for example, could lead to disturbed sleep and cause children to grab any scraps of sleep that they can; or perhaps sleep deprivation resulting in deeper sleep arriving more quickly and lasting for longer. These issues will also make someone less likely to wake up when they need a wee. While most children grow out of this, it may persist in some. I recently spoke to Neil, a graphic designer, about his son Kai's bedwetting. 'My wife and I both wet the bed until we were about 10, so it's not surprising that Kai is a bedwetter. However, he's 13 now and up until recently he was still wetting the bed every night.'

In the case of some children, bedwetting stops for a while only to reoccur. In these cases it is given the rather grand title of 'secondary enuresis' and may be due to something more concerning such as diabetes, which is why you should consult a doctor.

As to what to do about bedwetting, the key is for parents to avoid any sleep-deprived urge to be bad tempered and instead to do everything possible to save the child from embarrassment. After all, changing bed sheets at midnight is not such a huge deal for most of us. In contrast, the embarrassment that a child feels, or his/her avoidance of the good stuff of childhood, such as midnight feasts during sleepovers and school trips, is much more significant. This certainly rings true for Kai, who has rarely slept away from home due to his bedwetting. Neil explains: 'If there is a sleepover, my wife and I develop elaborate excuses to collect him at midnight. We might pretend that we are going away the next day at the crack of dawn.'

Neil continues: 'Recently, I pretty much forced him to go on a school trip, because I didn't want him to be the only kid in his year who was missing out. We made a plan before he left. I spoke to the teachers to ask that he was put in a room with some of the nicer kids. I also bought him five pairs of identical pyjamas so that he could throw one away each night if necessary. I gave him some pull-up padded pants too (even though some of the doctors we have spoken to don't recommend these). The plan was for him to wear these under his pyjamas without the other kids noticing. Unfortunately they did notice – which was mortifying for him.'

Neil is a kind and supportive parent, but not all parents take this thoughtful approach to a child's bedwetting. Some even punish children for their accidents, which is troublesome as parental punishment for bedwetting has been found to be associated with both depression in childhood and a poorer quality of life.[30] What is more, parents' attempts to stop unwanted bedwetting by using punishment may backfire and result in increasing its prevalence. Perhaps punishing bedwetting reflects a lack of understanding about the condition. In a survey of 216 parents, it was found that 26 per cent considered bedwetting to be due to laziness and 10 per cent to child defiance or behavioural problems.[31] This is concerning, given that neither is likely to have caused the bedwetting.

If bedwetting goes on, there are smart ways of dealing with it, and recently mobile phone apps have been developed to help bedwetters record a bladder diary documenting drinking and urination habits throughout the day and night.[32] There are also tips, such as making sure a child drinks a lot during the day and little in the evening. It's also possible for children to train their bladders, by drinking lots and then avoiding going to the toilet for a while. Alarms can be useful too. The pad and bell system involves putting a mat in the centre of the bed. If wetness is detected a bell goes off. This bell is out of reach of the child who must therefore get out of bed to turn it off, and at the same time should visit the toilet. The idea is that the brain eventually learns that a full bladder is a signal to wake up, so alertness is achieved before the urination begins. Reward charts can bring benefits, and children may be given a sticker or other treat on the nights that they have obtained dryness. This not only encourages dryness, but helps to keep track of progress. Drugs that reduce the amount of urine made by the kidneys can be prescribed in certain cases. In Kai's case, his dad tells me: 'We tried everything. We've had countless appointments about his bedwetting. Recently the doctor has prescribed a tricyclic antidepressant to be taken every night. This has allowed him to stay dry at night and I'm overjoyed to tell you that Kai has gone to stay with his cousins for a week. He wouldn't have dreamt of doing so a year ago, but the drug can have side-effects so we have to monitor the situation closely.'

Narcolepsy

Another sleep disorder that can bring challenges for the sufferer is narcolepsy. This is rare – thought to occur in around 25 to 50 people per 100,000.[33] Narcolepsy involves an irrepressible urge to fall asleep during the day. This isn't like the sleepiness that most of us experience from time to time, when at a mind-numbing meeting after lunch or watching a boxset before bed. This sleepiness is much more excessive and might involve falling asleep mid-sentence only a few hours into the day. It is often accompanied by cataplexy, which involves a sudden loss of muscle tone for anything from a number of seconds to a few minutes. This usually occurs in response to strong emotions such as anger, amusement or surprise. Someone might be arguing with a partner, laughing at a comedy show or unexpectedly spy a celebrity in the street and suddenly find that their muscles become weak. Perhaps their jaw will flop open or their head will roll forward. They might find that their knees give way and they take a tumble. The whole time they will be fully aware of this experience.

In many cases narcolepsy appears to be due to very low levels of the brain chemical hypocretin, which plays an important role in keeping us alert. These low levels of hypocretin likely reflect a loss of neurons in the hypothalamus, the area of the brain hosting the suprachiasmatic nucleus (SCN), which, as discussed in Chapter 1, is important for our 24-hour rhythm of sleep and wake. As to what causes this disorder, it appears to be an autoimmune disease, meaning that the immune system might be killing its own hypocretin-producing cells. The reasons why this happens are still being understood, but multiple genetic and environmental factors are likely to be important. Triggers can be as simple as catching the flu. In 2010, 54 children in Finland were diagnosed with narcolepsy.[34] While this may not sound like a lot of cases overall, this was startling as it represented a 17-fold increase compared with previous years. In trying to understand this unusual finding, it was discovered that 50 of the 54 children had received the Pandemrix vaccination against swine flu within the eight-month period before the onset of their narcolepsy. Perhaps the vaccination had contributed to the development of the disorder, together with other environmental influences and genetic vulnerability. So, both viral infections and a specific vaccination have been associated with narcolepsy, however overall risks remain very small. When I consider the advantages of immunisation and think about some of the consequences of missing out on vaccinations, such as the devastating effects of polio in my beloved Great Auntie Ethel, my own choice is to remain first in line to have myself and my children vaccinated.

For those suffering from this disorder, certain medications (including stimulants) and lifestyle adjustments can help. There are excellent support groups and websites* and it can be useful to learn that some of the symptoms are shared with those without narcolepsy too. These include sleep paralysis,

---

* For example, see www.narcolepsynetwork.org.

where it is not possible to move or speak for a short period just as the sufferer is falling asleep or waking up, and associated hallucinations. This symptom is so common in those with narcolepsy that, together with dream-like hallucinations, which occur during the onset of sleep (discussed in the next section), daytime sleepiness and cataplexy, it makes up the narcolepsy tetrad.

Sleep paralysis – a waking nightmare

In a 300-year-old cottage in the depths of the British countryside, Mrs Sinclair, aged 70 and living alone, awoke to find herself lying face down in her bed. She could feel hands around her neck, someone was throttling her. Somehow she managed to flip herself over to confront who she thought was a burglar. Instead she found a child-like imp laughing at her. He began pushing against her sides, tucking the bed sheets in around her. 'We've nearly strangled you and now we're tucking you in,' he goaded, in a way reminiscent of bullying children some 60 years previously. She tried to move but instead found herself 'tarmacked into the mattress', paralysed except for the ability to move her eyes. Although non-religious, the petrified Mrs Sinclair began mentally to recite the Lord's Prayer.

This might sound like the stuff of nightmares, but having researched sleep paralysis this story did not surprise me. Sleep paralysis involves being unable to move just as we are falling asleep or waking up and is often accompanied by hallucinations. Many people won't have heard of it, but it is intriguing. While pretty much all the research on this topic is focused on adults, sleep paralysis can occur at any age, so we should consider it along with the other sleep disorders covered in this chapter. We should take children seriously if they tell us that they were pinned to their bed and saw a ghost.

So what might have caused Mrs Sinclair's petrifying experience? Such experiences are often filed as paranormal. In Mrs Sinclair's case, she became convinced that her cottage was haunted. 'At one point I said to the ghost, "If you're stopping here, I want some rent off you,"' she told me. Similar things occurred every couple of months but she told nobody, fearing they would think she was 'demented'. The convergence of sleep research and paranormal psychology got me chatting about sleep paralysis over lunch with my aforementioned Goldsmiths colleague, French. He often appears on daytime TV shows such as *This Morning* to cast a sceptical eye over paranormal claims (and was even the resident sceptic on the ITV series *Haunted Homes*). He tells me he has lost count of the number of ghostly encounters that sounded to him like classic cases of sleep paralysis – an explanation that is usually rejected by the person making the claim. With my interest in sleep, it seemed ridiculous for us not to join forces and research the topic together.*

Paranormal explanations aside, how else might sleep paralysis be explained? Having had a similar experience in New Zealand when on holiday, Mrs Sinclair herself began to challenge her interpretation. 'Had the ghost followed me to New Zealand?' she wondered, before deciding that this was unlikely. This led her to search the internet, where she encountered sleep paralysis for the first time. She visited her doctor armed with this knowledge, but he rudely dismissed her, saying that he'd never heard of sleep paralysis.

This is when Mrs Sinclair contacted my colleague French, whom she had seen on the television. He explained that her experience was quite common and that during one of her episodes features of REM sleep, where the body is paralysed and dreams so commonly occur, spill over into waking life. French also sent Mrs Sinclair some of the papers we had worked on together.

One of these papers aimed to identify possible risk factors for sleep paralysis. For the study we asked more than 800 people (many of whom were twins) about the frequency with

---

* I would say it was 'fate' but being a signed-up member of the sceptics society, French would not approve. We have collaborated on this work with many others including Dr Brian Sharpless and Dr Dan Denis (mentioned in Chapter 1).

which they had experienced sleep paralysis.[35] We also asked them about other things that might be linked to this paralysis, such as anxiety, the quality of their sleep, caffeine use and smoking.

Overall, we found that roughly a third of our participants reported experiencing sleep paralysis at least once in their lives. This percentage was higher than expected, but estimates from different studies tend to vary quite extensively. We also found that poor sleep quality, anxiety symptoms and threatening life events were all associated with sleep paralysis. While our study did not show that these things caused sleep paralysis (or vice versa), it would be interesting to try to understand through future research exactly why there are these associations.

We then compared the twins in our study to try to understand more about genetic and environmental risks for sleep paralysis. We found that identical twins were more similar in their reports of whether they had experienced sleep paralysis than non-identical twins. We used this information to estimate that there is moderate genetic influence on sleep paralysis. From our study, it seemed that genetic and environmental influences appeared to be more or less equally important in explaining why people differ in their experiences of sleep paralysis.

After highlighting the importance of genes in sleep paralysis, we examined some specific genes that have been previously linked to different aspects of our slumber and the body clock. We found an interesting association with a genetic variant in the PER2 gene.* This has previously been associated with our diurnal preference – the extent to which we are a morning- or evening-type person – and with aspects of sleep, such as quality. We were excited to be among the

---

* Our results should be considered preliminary as our sample was particularly small. Furthermore, our molecular genetic results were not statistically significant after accounting for the fact that we also looked at a number of other genetic variants. This finding could be due to chance and needs to be replicated using much larger samples.

first to examine this important topic. Taking the field as a whole, it seems that stress and anything that disrupts the sleep cycle could increase the chances of someone experiencing sleep paralysis and this emphasises the value of a consistent sleep routine yet again.

When I asked Mrs Sinclair if she still believes that there is a ghost in her house she replied without hesitation: 'Definitely not! My experiences were stress-related. I've had a lot going on over the past few years.' Mrs Sinclair has not had an episode of sleep paralysis since her discussion with French, so does not yet know if this new information will be helpful during an episode. However, she still feels relieved: 'I now know it's not going to kill me. I feel very, very, very fortunate to have spoken to Professor French.'

To further help people like Mrs Sinclair, we need to understand whether techniques that have been shown to be effective in relaxing us and aiding good sleep, such as mindfulness, could also have a knock-on effect in reducing sleep paralysis. We need to know not just who is likely to experience episodes, but when they are likely to occur. We want to develop methods to prevent these experiences, or to help people cope with them. We want them to be less frightening – although interestingly some sufferers report feeling no fear at all.

Indeed, another person I spoke to explained that when she'd first had an episode she was on a train, next to her mother. She didn't know what was happening to her, but had never considered being fearful. Instead, she felt comforted to have her mother by her side. She has managed to retain this feeling of comfort during episodes ever since. Others have reported finding sleep paralysis blissful or have even filed it away as a positive supernatural experience. Understanding why people react so differently to this inability to move might provide information that we can use to help sufferers be less frightened by their experiences.

Research on this topic is really in its infancy, and for sufferers it can be reassuring simply to know that this common experience has a name, that they are not alone in having

episodes and that sleep paralysis often runs in families.*
Shortly after our paper was reported in the press, we received
an email from someone who had read about our research in
the *Huffington Post*. He had experienced sleep paralysis for
much of his life and his father and his sister had also reported
episodes. He ended his email by writing: 'This may not be at
all relevant to you, but today is the first day we've had a name
and description for what was/is going on, and we're relieved ...
and I just had to thank someone.'

Anecdotally, it seems that sleep paralysis occurs in children:
some children find themselves in a petrified state, awake but
unable to move. But what research is there on this topic?
There is a lack of it examining this systematically in young
children, however there is a little focusing on adolescents. In
high schools in Mexico City it was found that over a quarter
of those questioned had experienced sleep paralysis (an
experience referred to in the study as 'a dead body climbed
on top of me' – accompanied by an inability to move or
speak).[36] This topic needs to be systematically researched at
different stages of life so that perhaps the reassuring messages
beginning to reach adult sufferers can reach our children
too.

Exploding head syndrome

'Mostly it's a "guitar" strings sound, as if an electric guitar is
plugged in and a large object falls on the strings...'
'The explosions ... they are just like that, yes. Like a gun ...
more electric though, like lightning. It seems to hurt but
doesn't. Only wakes me up. However, I am terrified, my
adrenaline races through my entire body and my heart feels
like it just stops. It's like being bucked off a horse.
Terrifying...'

---

* There are also some psychological and pharmacological treatment
options, but there is not yet strong data to support these.

These are real descriptions by those who experience another poorly publicised sleep problem. It's called exploding head syndrome. You read that correctly. This might sound like a term used in a sensational newspaper headline, but it's a real sleep disorder.

Despite my long-standing interest in sleep, I first heard about this syndrome from my aforementioned workmate French, who sent an email to all his colleagues, asking if anyone was interested in meeting Dr Brian Sharpless, an associate professor at the American School of Professional Psychology at Argosy University, Northern Virginia. He also happens to be author of *Unusual and Rare Psychological Disorders*[37] and is the world expert in this syndrome. After spending a few minutes musing over other body parts exploding (could there be a flying eye syndrome too?) I wrote back to jump at the opportunity.

Within a week I was sitting face to face with Sharpless and hearing all about this fascinating disorder. Noticing my bemusement at the name of the disorder, he told me: 'Exploding head syndrome may have the best name in medicine, but it's a bit misleading because the head doesn't actually explode. That would be a really bad disorder. It certainly gets attention from the public, but [Sharpless' colleague Professor] Peter Goadsby and I have argued to change the name to "episodic cranial sensory shocks" in order to make it sound less hyperbolic and to draw attention to the fact that people can also experience visual effects during episodes (for example, seeing light flashes or TV static). Disorders, like some rock stars, need a name change as they get older and more mature.'

Sharpless went on to tell me more about the disorder, which involves perceiving a loud noise or flash of light upon falling asleep or waking up.[38] This might be similar to seeing a bolt of lightning or hearing a firework, but there is no external cause. It's not just a car backfiring outside or a shelf falling down that causes this – I asked. It wakes us up pretty quickly and can be frightening and upsetting. However, it's also pretty benign and doesn't cause pain. Having said that, anyone concerned should visit a doctor, who may want to rule out more concerning disorders such as epilepsy.

As to what causes this odd occurrence, the jury is out – although I'm currently collaborating on a number of projects aimed at answering this question. Perhaps the leading current theory is that the usual process of falling asleep is disturbed. Typically, as we fall asleep, the reticular formation in the brain stem starts to inhibit our ability to move, see, and hear things. In the case of exploding head syndrome, it has been proposed that, instead of shutting down the auditory neurons, it actually causes them to fire all at once. This is what gives those characteristic 'bangs'. As Sharpless described, not everyone agrees with this explanation. He told me: 'Some of the more interesting emails I've received were from people with exploding head syndrome. Some would tell me how foolish I was for believing the "medical explanations" when they know it's caused by cell phones, active utility monitoring systems, or nefarious government agents. For them, it is microwaves being directed at their heads which causes these explosions, not a blip in normal sleep processes.'

Most people who have had this experience are not concerned, but some are. Sharpless went on to explain: 'I've worked with some people who experience episodes five to seven times each night. For them, it is a real burden. Fortunately, in the studies I've done, only about 15 per cent of the people who experience exploding head syndrome are negatively affected by it.' For those who are, there are unfortunately few tried-and-tested treatments – although it's been proposed that any technique aimed at reducing stress might be helpful.

When I ask Sharpless about these experiences in children, it seems that, again, we know little. 'We don't know very much about isolated sleep paralysis in kids, and even less about exploding head syndrome,' he said. But he's onto it and suggested a future collaboration in order to learn more.

Help!

It's clear that children, and adults too for that matter, can experience a huge number of sleep difficulties and disorders – of which only a small proportion are discussed here. Given the frequency of these sleep problems, many people are looking for help. So what is out there? Doctors should be the first port of call – but many will have had limited training in sleep medicine. So what other advice is available? There are excellent books written for clinicians on paediatric sleep such as *A Clinical Guide to Pediatric Sleep: Diagnosis and management of sleep problems* (mentioned previously, and which is drawn upon in some of the advice given in this chapter);[20] and *Pediatric Sleep Problems: A Clinician's Guide to Behavioral Interventions*.[39] Caregivers struggling with sleep difficulties in children might also be interested in *Solve Your Child's Sleep Problems*[40] and *Solving Children's Sleep Problems: A step-by-step guide for parents*.[41] Some books are heavily designed for use with children, such as *What to Do When You Dread Your Bed*.[42] Websites and phone apps have been designed to deal specifically with children's sleep problems. Some have been developed by impressive sleep researchers from leading hospitals. Studies need to examine the effectiveness of these apps, but they have great potential.

We should feel that we can question our doctors too. Why is it that most of us seem more comfortable asking questions about the inner workings of a used car than we do of our own bodies? Doctors sometimes prescribe drugs but can be unwilling to engage in any discussion about their thought process or the reasoning behind decisions. Could it be that behavioural treatments are preferable, as seems to be the case for so many sleep problems?* When prescribing

---

* Although, not for some sleep disorders such as narcolepsy and sleep apnoea.

drugs, possible side-effects are sometimes not discussed. This may be particularly noteworthy for melatonin – a naturally occurring hormone that is considered by many experts to be beneficial to certain children.[43] It's also popular with parents who sometimes perceive it to be 'natural' and effective in reducing sleep problems in their children.[44] Nonetheless, it has been pointed out that studies haven't really followed up with children who have been prescribed this drug over long periods of time to check how safe it is, and it is not registered for use in children.[45] Then there are concerns about the contents of melatonin pills when bought without a prescription. In a study of supplements bought over the counter in Canada, it was found that the concentration of melatonin in pills ranged from 83 per cent less than that stated on the package – to an alarming 478 per cent more.[46] The chemical serotonin was also found in 8 of the 31 samples assessed, which is concerning, as when consumed in large quantities it can be dangerous. Overall, we have to feel free to question advice and follow what we think is right for us. That goes for any tips provided in this book.

It's also good to remember the transient nature of childhood. What seems unbearable one day is not a problem the next. While bedtime struggles or sleeplessness can persist over time[47] and can bring entire families (plus long-suffering neighbours) to their knees, problems come and go. This was illustrated nicely by looking at data from a study in Australia. Parents of over 4,000 children were asked about how their children sleep. Quite a lot of parents (13 per cent) reported their children to have moderate or severe sleep problems when they were aged four to five years old. When asked about their children's sleep just two years later, more than three-quarters of the parents who had previously considered their child to have a moderate or severe sleep disorder no longer considered this to be the case.[48]

Just go to sleep!

All in all, the sleep challenges accompanying the earliest stages of life typically reduce as children grow up and start sleeping through the night. But with development, children may be more likely to experience other problems. A shift in sleep architecture, such as the decrease in REM sleep, makes certain problems more likely. An increased understanding of the world, together with skill development such as learning to read, can mean that some children emerge from their emotional cocoon to experience anxieties that make it difficult for them to sleep. Improved communication skills allow children to tell us about things that might have happened during the night, of which we were once blissfully unaware. So instead of thinking *just go to sleep* we should perhaps listen carefully and if necessary explain that there is a perfectly reasonable explanation for having seen that ghost.

CHAPTER FOUR

Laaazzzy? Adolescents' Sleep

Teenagers (13–18 years) recommended 8–10 hours of sleep per 24 hours[1]

Are adolescents as lazy as they sometimes seem?

In the early 1990s, aged 14, I became obsessed with a hi-fi system in my local high street electronics shop. It excited me so much that it kept me awake at night: a Sony creation with a double cassette player, a CD drawer and a record player on top. To my teenage self it represented both the height of technological sophistication and something that would be the coolest status symbol. The only issue was the huge amount of money I would have to save in order to purchase the beast.

Too young to work in a shop, I took on a paper round, lugging a huge sack of newspapers around my neighbourhood. And because the good folk of St Margarets in south-west London wanted to read their papers while still chowing down their breakfasts, my new job involved me waking before 6 a.m. I achieved this for a while – and being one of the few females on the round, I acquired two suitors who would come on their bikes to help me out, following the completion of their own paper rounds. But, with time, the conflict between my adolescent sleep requirements and my desire to once a week squirrel away 16 of Her Majesty's finest pounds for my hi-fi became too much.

I ended up lying in bed begging my mum to take over for the day. And being the kind-hearted, socially minded person that she is, unable to stand the thought of the shopkeeper or paper-readers being let down – Mum would trundle around the streets with my bag of newspapers. She still finds it amusing to recall the shock of my suitors at seeing her lugging the paper bag (plus she's still slightly put out that they never offered to help).

Most of us recognise this sort of teenage behaviour – and a tale such as this tends to make adolescents seem lazy. The truth is, however, that people at this age are dealing heroically with the most overwhelming physiological and social changes, simply trying to navigate this difficult period of life.

So why do adolescents find an early start such a big deal? Well, in short, it's because it is a big deal for them. In fact, it's a huge deal. If you ask an adolescent to get up at 6 a.m., whether to deliver papers or get to school on time, you're putting the same pressure on their bodies as if you asked a younger child, or adult, to rise much earlier – at, say, 4 a.m. Their bodies are better suited to being fast asleep.

We know this from studies of melatonin levels. Melatonin is the darkness hormone discussed in Chapter 2 and that the body makes most profusely during the middle of the night. When you compare melatonin levels in adolescents with those in people of other ages, the peak of this hormone occurs later in adolescents. This effectively suggests that the biological clock delays, or shifts later, at this stage of life compared with others – and it would help to explain why adolescents go to bed late and struggle to get up in the morning.

But what causes this shift in melatonin dynamics and the associated late bedtime and wake time in adolescents? This phase delay, as it's called, has long been attributed to adolescents having far too much going on to go to bed early. They have homework to finish, jobs to do, parties to attend and now numerous social media sites to monitor for fear of missing out on any social news. They work hard and they play hard. On top of this, parents start to give them greater autonomy in deciding when they go to bed. Together, these factors mean that their bedtimes become late, then later, and their body clock and melatonin levels eventually fall into line with their apparent behavioural choices.

But, upon deeper inspection, the situation appears to be much more complex than this.[2] In particular, the onrush of biological change that is puberty seems much more important than chronological age alone. For example, it's been found that the more physically developed teenagers are the later they like to go to bed. The research points to changes in sleep patterns being another consequence of the extraordinary hormonal changes that take place during adolescence.

It's too bright

Scientists have wracked their brains to try and work out what exactly might be causing the phase delay in adolescents. What could be going on to make so many of them sleep at such unusual times? These sleep patterns seem to largely occur regardless of where teenagers live and what they like doing. Bedtime appears to become later during adolescence whether they are based in New Zealand,[3] Japan,[4] Finland[5] or elsewhere, and regardless of whether cultures are pre- or post-industrial.[6] This shift is even found in other mammals too.

One prominent idea to explain this delay has focused on light. Because light is the most important factor for syncing the internal 24-hour circadian clock with the surrounding world, it's been thought that changes in a person's sensitivity to light at different stages of life could be important. It's been proposed that youths might become more sensitive to evening light as they get older. If the evening felt lighter to them, they might feel more wakeful, something that could mess with their ability to fall asleep early. In a neat experiment, scientists from the US tested this hypothesis by exposing adolescents to light at different stages of puberty. They looked at how their bodies responded in terms of their melatonin secretion.[7] The team expected that the more developed the adolescent, the more sensitive they would be to light in the evening and the more their spike in melatonin release would be suppressed. It would therefore take longer for them to receive the cue that their bodies need to go to sleep and bedtime would push later. Intriguingly, contrary to expectations they found quite the reverse. The less-developed adolescents were the most sensitive to light in the evening. This led the researchers to revise their hypothesis. They suggested instead that the phase delay might be caused by older adolescents having greater exposure to light rather than them being more sensitive to it per se. Perhaps older adolescents have more freedom and are more likely to spend their evenings watching TV or surfing the web, or just generally being in well-lit environments than younger ones. This might suggest that behavioural choice as well as changes based on fundamental biology are important. Overall, it might be that as children enter puberty their increased sensitivity to light kicks off the process that delays the body clock, which results in a later bedtime and behavioural changes that lead to increased evening light exposure.

It's been a long day

Another proposal for this timing shift focuses on the idea that the pace of our body clock might change at different stages of life. Naturally, the internal human clock runs for a period of approximately 24 hours. But there is certainly a case of different folks having different (clock) strokes – and the internal day varies from one person to another. To account for the unique sleep timing found during adolescence, it's been suggested that as an adolescent gets older, his or her 'internal day' might get longer. Such a shift is intuitively appealing, and it would neatly account for a desire to go to bed progressively later, but gaining experimental support for it presented challenges.

One might wonder how on earth we can assess the pace of an internal clock given that it is constantly being adjusted by zeitgebers – or rather aspects of the environment such as light, which help to synchronise the internal body clock with the world around us. Indeed, it can be tricky. We could get very useful information on how fast adolescents' body clocks ticked if we were allowed to lock a bunch of them up in pitch-black caves, with no contact with anyone or anything that could mess with their internal clocks. But I'm not sure that would be very nice and ethics committees would never allow it. Instead, researchers have developed other techniques that tweak our experiences of the world to find out about the natural speed of our clocks. One technique is called 'forced desynchrony'. This typically involves inviting someone to a laboratory and giving them a different pattern of light and dark than they would normally experience. The important thing here is that the 'artificial day' has to be made substantially shorter or longer than expected (by several hours), otherwise the body would adapt to the new light schedule and we wouldn't be able to measure what was really going on. So, participants might be put on 20- or 28-hour cycles, with lights on for around a third of the day and lights off for the rest.

Such investigations are necessarily conducted in windowless laboratories that give nothing away about what time it is in the outside world. I was able to visit a participant involved in a similar type of experiment while I was working at a sleep laboratory in Pennsylvania. On the condition that I gave away zero clues as to the actual time of day or night, I was allowed a glimpse at his world. Upon entering the small bedroom in which this man was spending the week, I glanced around at the guitar, pile of books and the running machine that he'd been given to pass the time with. I'd arrived after a long day of work and was tired. I was ready to relax into the evening, my body slowly coasting towards bedtime – but he thought it was the early morning.

I didn't really trust myself not to yawn or to suddenly blurt out that I had to leave to go to bed, so I kept my conversation painfully stilted. His initially clear eagerness for company quickly turned to boredom. Given the choice to chat with the surprisingly dull Doctor G from London or continue his regimented lab life instead, he chose the latter. It was kind of awkward watching him look for excuses to tie up the conversation when he didn't have places to go or people to see. He couldn't even claim to need to see a man about a dog.

Forced desynchrony studies allow researchers to estimate a person's intrinsic day length because a 28-hour day, for example, is simply too long for the subject's body clock to snap into line. The researchers measure various physiological parameters to infer what time their bodies think it is. For example, they might focus on two things that are controlled by the inner clock (which are typically referred to as the clock 'outputs'): the darkness hormone melatonin and core body temperature.

It's now probably pretty obvious why they focus on melatonin – few things point so reliably to where the hands of our body clock are pointing than the pattern of this hormone's secretion. Because melatonin is typically produced by the body during the evening when darkness sets in (peaking later during the night), researchers avoid the possibility that light could mess with the melatonin secretion, by assessing it in dim-light conditions.

Another output scientists focus on is core body temperature because in the same way that melatonin release is predictable, the internal body clock also exerts a stereotypical control over our body temperature. The changes are slight – and we never deviate very far from our average 37°C – but we are warmest in the evening and coolest in the early hours of the morning and some hours before we habitually wake.

In a study reported in 1999, researchers in the USA invited 10 adolescents, aged on average 13 and a half, to live in the laboratory for around two weeks in an attempt to assess their intrinsic rhythms.[8] The participants spent their days on a schedule, which involved fun activities such as crafts in the afternoons and watching films in the evening. Their lives were shifted to run on 28-hour cycles, and their salivary melatonin and body temperature were monitored at various times.

The researchers found that every single adolescent in their study had an internal day of longer than 24 hours – with an average clock period of 24.3 hours. This may not sound particularly dramatic, but the authors suggested it might be slightly longer than that normally reported in adults.[*] The authors took this to support the original suggestion that perhaps the internal day is longer for adolescents than for

---

[*] Which is more like 24.1 when assessed using similar methods.[6]

other age groups. Consistent evidence comes from a study of male rats, which similarly found developmental changes in circadian rhythms,[9] although it has been argued that the change reported in the latter study might not have been related to puberty. Overall it is not currently entirely clear whether the body clock period lengthens during adolescence and in doing so contributes to a shift in sleep timing.

Not feeling sleepy?

A final theory to be considered that has been proposed to explain the changes in sleep timing during adolescence focuses on 'sleep homeostasis'. The concept of sleep homeostasis, as you may remember from Chapter 1, stems from work showing that the longer an animal is awake, the greater its sleep drive. Regarding adolescents, it has been proposed that as humans turn this developmental corner, they have to be awake for longer periods in order to feel sleepy. So, whereas children may be exhausted and fall asleep quickly if they go to bed at 11 p.m., this might be trickier for adolescents because they simply haven't been awake for long enough to feel sleepy yet. It then makes sense that as adolescents become more developed they put themselves to bed a little later.

Support for this idea comes from a study by scientists in the USA.[10] They invited a group of children and adolescents to visit their laboratory. Around half of them hadn't yet started puberty: they were in that in-between stage of around 11 years of age – on the cusp of leaving childhood behind and becoming adolescents. The other half were more developed: they were around 13 years old and their bodies were starting to resemble those of adults. The researchers asked all the participants to stay up for 36 hours while sitting in bed wired up to a polysomnogram – a system that measures brainwaves and other physiological variables to accurately detect if you are asleep or not. Every two hours the youths were told to sit quietly, keep their eyes closed and try to fall asleep – and they were given 20 minutes to try to do this. Lovely, you'd think. However, if they did fall asleep they were woken up. The experience might have been similar to trying to get some kip on a plane when sitting next to someone who has been a bit too enthusiastic about the inflight bar.

The researchers were interested in whether the youths managed to fall asleep and if so, how long it took them to do so. The quicker they fell asleep (and, of course, *if* they fell asleep), the greater the sleep homeostasis mechanism was inferred to be driving the participants to sleep.

Early in the evening, at around 8.30 p.m., there was no difference between the child and adolescent groups. However, later in the evening, from 10.30 p.m. (14.5 hours since they'd last slept) until 2.30 a.m., they found that the children were more likely to fall asleep and did so more quickly than the adolescents. So, just as originally expected, it seems that adolescents need to be awake for longer than children in order to get sleepy and fall asleep, a theory that has been supported by other studies.[11]

Looking at the huge amount of research conducted over the years, it seems that lots of different processes interact to result in what has been referred to as the 'perfect storm'.[12] Adolescents do not feel sleepy at a typical bedtime and so go to bed later and later; and light perhaps does an insufficient job to help them adjust to a schedule driven by society and social factors. This all results in a hell of a problem getting up in the morning.

Why did teenage owls evolve?

As we begin to understand what is causing adolescents to behave like owls, we are left wondering: what sort of evolutionary advantage could there be in allowing adolescents to run out of sync with everyone else in society? Intuitively, this would seem likely to impede their integration into the community and potentially lead to conflict and harm. Researchers sometimes talk about evolutionary reasons why adolescents distance themselves from their families and affiliate with their peers.[13] Perhaps, if adolescents are on a similar schedule to one another, which differs from the schedules of others, this process is facilitated? Perhaps if they are the only ones awake and functioning on their specific schedule, they are the only ones to hang out with? Or having adolescents awake at night could have allowed them to protect the herd. This might have been particularly valuable in years gone by. If we sleep on different schedules at different stages of our lives, then we can all take a turn in staying awake to watch over the group.[14] Sleep makes us vulnerable, so having someone awake at any one time could increase survival and have evolutionary advantages. Adolescents, who are young and strong, take what is likely to be the most dangerous shift: night-time.

This specific sleep timing may also have evolved to provide adolescents with a greater opportunity to be awake at night – a time during which romantic encounters are most common.[15] Nighttime also brings less competition from older members of the group, so finding a mate may be easier. This pattern might have also encouraged greater autonomy and independence at this pivotal point in human development.

But not all adolescents like a lie-in!

But what about those adolescents who are members of a rowing club and bound effortlessly out of bed at 5 a.m. every morning? Does this disprove the adolescent change in sleep timing? Not at all. When presenting a scientific argument to non-scientists they sometimes point to an exception to 'disprove' a statement. 'Smoking causes cancer' can lead to 'my nan smoked 40 a day for 80 years and lived until she was 100'. In these discussions the sceptic is missing the point. Nobody is claiming that everyone who smokes will become ill. Instead, we are often referring to an association. So, instead of all smoking grandmothers getting cancer, we are saying something quite different. If you have two clubs full of nans and one club is exclusively for smokers and the other is for non-smokers – whereas perhaps 12 per cent of the smokers could receive a lung cancer diagnosis, this may be just 1 per cent in the latter group.

Those genetic differences

Just as it can be pointed out that not all smoking nans get cancer, it can be noted that not all adolescents go to bed late or struggle to get up in the morning. There are endless examples of teenagers who bust the rules and have a hard time staying up late. These differences between adolescents are important, as those who are evening types may experience more difficulties than others. For example, in a study of over 2,000 adolescents aged 12–18 years old, it was found that being a night owl was linked to poorer self-regulation, such as forgetting instructions easily or behaving impulsively.[16] Other studies have also reported links between having an evening preference and multiple other things, including increased sensation-seeking, binge-drinking, substance use and aggressive behaviour.[17-19]

As for what explains the difference between people in terms of preferred timing, genes and the environment remain important. As for which genes are likely to play a role, a handful of candidates have been explored. These include the 'clock genes' or 'circadian genes', such as *CLOCK*, *PER1*, *PER2* and *PER3*. Different people have different versions of these genes and those with certain types are more likely to function best in the morning. It's not that someone could look at your DNA and know for sure whether you prefer to get up early or stay up late. Instead, it's possible that if an appropriately skilled lab technician had DNA from a group of 10,000 people who were morning types and 10,000 who were evening types, they could tell which DNA samples came from which group. Certain versions of genes would be expected to crop up more often in one group than the other.

One 'clock gene' in which there has been a lot of interest is a variation in *PER3*. Humans are genetically very similar and only differ in very small ways. It's normal for sections of our DNA to be repeated, and one way that we can vary from one another is in terms of how many times certain parts are repeated. For *PER3*, a specific section of DNA is either repeated four or five times. This difference has been related to when we like to do things, and those with five repeats are more likely to be morning types than those with four repeats.[*] We don't really know why this is. However, it is likely that this genetic difference affects the amount and type of protein made by the *PER3* gene, which could in turn affect our internal body clock.[21] Discussing this with Simon Archer, professor of molecular biology at the University of Surrey, he tells me: 'The repeat sequence variation in *PER3* appears to be specific to primates and may have evolved to allow them to be more adapted to a diurnal lifestyle. Because it is also associated with different diurnal preference, morning preference or evening preference, this could have helped early social individual humans to be active and alert at different times of day, enhancing survival.' So, just as adolescents work on a slightly altered time schedule from others in society, people with four repeats of the *PER3* polymorphism may be on a slightly different schedule to those with five repeats.

It is pretty clear that the many quirky differences between us, such as when we like to wake up, the time we perform best at work or sport and when we prefer to turn in for the night, are affected by multiple genes, each of which plays a small role in explaining these differences between us. As mentioned previously (see Chapter 2), this knowledge has resulted in researchers upping the ante and focusing on a huge number of genetic differences between us (running genome-wide association studies). Recent studies of this type have been reassuring in revealing that, as expected, morning preference is associated with lots of genetic variants near the clock genes (including, for example, the legendary *PER3*).[22,23]

TV to watch! No time for sleep

Moving on from genetics and considering which aspects of the environment could contribute to differences in the time

---

[*] In our own work, led by Nicola Barclay of the University of Oxford, we did not manage to replicate this particular association in a small study.[20]

we go to sleep, many influences are likely to be involved. Some of these are discussed elsewhere, such as the consumption of too much caffeine, which is not only found in coffee but in various products, including energy drinks. Indeed, afternoon and evening caffeine use has been found to delay the body clock[24] and alcohol might have a similar influence.[25] There has recently been a focus on electronic media use in adolescence too. The reason for this is twofold. First of all, it doesn't take a scientist to notice that electronics are everywhere – we're all at it. Even the reluctant get sucked in. The numbers are quite shocking. This was shown in a 2006 study by the National Sleep Foundation, an impressive organisation in the USA, designed in part to educate the public about the importance of 40 winks for their health and safety. Researchers called up more than 1,600 parents and carers of adolescents. They asked them which electronic items could be found in their children's bedrooms.[26] Perhaps alarmingly, almost all (97 per cent!) of the children had at least one electronic item in their room. Most typically they had an electronic music device, but more than 50 per cent had a TV and almost half had a mobile phone.* Having all of this stuff lying about can mean that there is just no time to sleep – and if there is time, children are just too pumped up to be able to bunk down for the night.[28] To understand more about how technology might affect sleep, the National Sleep Foundation conducted a further poll in 2011, which focused on technology use and sleep in 13- to 64-year-olds.[29] They found that 96 per cent of those who were younger than 30 years old used technology in the hour before bed (with 72 per cent of adolescents using their mobile phone during this period).

The second reason why electronic media use has been the focus of research concerns the glow emitted from certain

---

* A more recent survey conducted in 2014 by the National Sleep Foundation found that 75 per cent of children had at least one technological device in their bedroom. Having devices on after bedtime was associated with poorer sleep quality.[27]

products. While 'electronic media' encompasses a whole range of things (including music players, video consoles and computers), certain examples, such as mobile phones and tablets, can be particularly problematic because of the type of light they emit. Light comes in different colours depending on its wavelength. The light that we can see ranges from violet, which has the shortest wavelength, to red, with the longest. Towards the shortest wavelength end of the visible spectrum is blue light. This is the type of light we see outside on a beautiful summer's day and is also the kind emitted by many phones and tablets. But here lies a problem. This is the type of light that has the potential to be most damaging to our sleep. Light is key in synchronising our internal clock to the outside world and determining when the darkness hormone, melatonin, is released by our bodies. So, next time we look at our phones or tablets before bed, we should keep in mind that we are effectively telling our bodies that it is daytime. We are instructing our body to hold off releasing melatonin, which is why we might not feel sleepy. Over and above, there is research to suggest that light is acutely alerting and has a direct effect on our brain even independently of the circadian system.[30] Not only does electronic media use delay our sleep, but it may also affect other aspects of our slumber, resulting in overall shorter sleep, for example.[28] Electronic media is problematic at other times of life too, and it's been revealed that babies and toddlers who use touchscreens daily sleep less than others. In fact, one study found that they slept for 15.6 minutes less for each additional hour using the tablet.[31]

As to what to do about this, the obvious answer is that we should avoid electronic media before bedtime. The National Sleep Foundation has recommended that we turn off all electronic devices at least an hour before bedtime. Apparently Harvard Medical School has suggested avoiding exposure to blue light a full two to three hours before bedtime.[32] Another suggestion is that we limit the duration of time spent exposed to blue light before we plan to head to the land of nod. Some studies have found that exposure to just one hour of screen time is perhaps not enough to affect our melatonin or sleep in a clinically significant way.[33,34] However, overall, it seems that the longer we are exposed to bright light, the greater our melatonin suppression and the more our timing is shifted.[35,*] Scientists do not agree on exactly how long is too long. But the overall message is clear: if you insist on spending time with your electronics before bed, limit it.

For those of us who can't resist a cheeky late-night tweet or gossip with our chums via WhatsApp, orange-tinted glasses have been designed to avoid the impact of blue light on our eyes.[36] For those reticent to don a pair, perhaps seeing them fashioned by will.i.am or Bono might help to seal the deal. But glasses aside, perhaps best of all, researchers have been heckling the big companies to deal with this issue. Tech giants like Apple and Amazon have finally acknowledged the problem and made changes to the light emission of some of their products at night. Many phones can now be set to a night mode, to produce a less disruptive and more alluring-sounding, red-orange light.[37] Given the significance of good quality sleep for so many aspects of our lives, and the extent of our use of mobile phones and tablets, this must have been a fist-pumping moment for the sleep researchers involved in this change. Let's just hope this hard work doesn't backfire and these light changes become used as an excuse to tweet, WhatsApp and work late into the night. Instead, it might be useful to limit our use of technology, such as by adopting the 'no email outside of work' policy, or buying a family lockbox, where everyone can deposit their smartphones to charge before bed.[38]

Ignoring your phone or changing the light it emits may still not be enough. It's better to take electronic devices out of the bedroom altogether. In a review of the association between mobile phones/tablets and sleep in over 125,000 children

---

* Interestingly, it has also been found that shorter durations of light exposure have a greater impact on the circadian rhythm and melatonin when the effect is considered per minute.[35]

between 6 and 19 years of age, it was found that devices in the bedroom, even when not being used, can disrupt sleep.[39] We don't want to go to sleep wondering whether responses to important emails may ding while we are catching our Zs, or be tempted to check messages when we wake up in the night. Just as when we're considering whether to add that triple-fudge chocolate cake to our shopping basket, it's best to avoid temptation. Understanding why some teenagers can switch off their phones and other technology without a fuss, whereas others struggle to part with their devices, is an important topic for researchers as we move forward.

Epigenetics: above the genome

As we scramble to understand the complexities of genetic and environmental influences on our sleep-timing preferences, along comes epigenetics (which means 'above genetics') to add a layer of complexity. You may have heard of epigenetics in the popular press. In a nutshell, we've known for a long time that the sequence of DNA we are born with stays as good as identical over our entire lives and is important in helping to make us who we are. This DNA sequence is the same in pretty much every cell in our body. What is more novel is a research focus on epigenetics, which addresses how we can turn our genes on and off, or turn them down, a bit like using a dimmer switch, when we don't need them to do their thing. Epigenetic influences are dynamic, meaning that they can be influenced by the environment – such as whether we are smokers or not. They also vary during our lives, and adolescence is thought to be a particularly interesting time for epigenetic changes given what we know about other physical changes taking place across this period. One way that epigenetics works is by a process referred to as 'DNA methylation'. 'Methyl groups' (carbon and hydrogen compounds) can bind to our DNA so that it can no longer deliver its message or the number of audible words is altered.[40] Let's think of DNA as a mouth and methyl as a sock. If someone sticks a sock in your mouth, you won't be able to express anything profound, no matter what your potential for elegant communication. Of course this analogy over-simplifies things and actually much of what is going on at the molecular level remains a mystery. So, we may well have genes that make us more or less likely to function well during the evening – but the extent to which they are turned on or off is probably just as important.

In trying to understand more about how epigenetics may be important for diurnal preference, I was involved in a project where I worked with epigenetic researchers Dr Chloe Wong and Dr Emma Dempster. We focused on a small sample of identical twins who differed from one another in terms of their preference for daily activities and their sleep timing.[41] We considered identical twins because we know that differences between them are not due to their genes (they are genetic clones). Instead, it is possible that epigenetic differences between them can help to explain variations in their sleep-timing preferences. In other words, maybe there was something different about the environment of each twin and this was affecting how their DNA was expressed. We focused on genome-wide patterns of DNA methylation, meaning that we looked at DNA methylation differences between these twins across all of their DNA. We were excited to see methylation differences between those who preferred to function at different times. It seemed that epigenetic differences between identical twins could help to explain why one might prefer to go to bed and wake up earlier than the other.* As we move forward, we need to understand which environmental differences can affect gene expression and have an impact on sleep.

Social jetlag

Moving back to the general change in sleep timing that occurs in adolescence leads us to consider social jetlag. While

---

* Of note, there are other possible explanations for these results. Overall, it was fascinating to work on this project, and learn from some terrific epigeneticists, but while we have perhaps helped to get the ball rolling in this research area, bigger and better studies remain the future.

this may sound like the pastime *de rigueur* for adolescence, it is nothing of the sort. Social jetlag often occurs from living a life that is discrepant from what our biology is requesting. For example, the bodies of adolescents may be screaming at them to go to bed at midnight and to get up after 9 a.m. In reality, school start times dictate that they need to try to get to bed earlier, although homework, sports and other school activities get in the way. They might then have to wake up at 6 a.m. At the weekend, social pressures and making up for the sleep loss from the school week may mean that they are staying up late and then sleeping until noon. Sleeping in over the weekend delays the body clock.[42] These fluctuations in sleep timing result in a loss of synchrony between internal clocks and the external world, and can lead to a constant feeling of jetlag. When Sunday night rocks up, teens essentially have to navigate back multiple time zones in order to cope with their Monday morning rise time. This is particularly problematic as it can take some time to adjust to jetlag, so just as adolescents are beginning to get used to their early start, along comes the weekend – and timings shift yet again.

And just when we thought things couldn't get any worse, it's been pointed out that not only does each week start with jetlag, but with the worst type of jetlag, where we need to go to bed and get up earlier than we did previously.[43] This is just like flying eastwards (from San Francisco to New York, rather than from New York to San Francisco). What is more, it has now been proposed that social jetlag could be associated with a whole heap of undesirables, such as smoking, drinking alcohol and suffering from depression.[44] Indeed, in a recent study it was found that among US high school students, social jetlag predicted subsequent heavy drinking.[25] Social jetlag has also been associated with lower brain response to reward.[45] This might suggest that when experiencing social jetlag adolescents need to up the ante on the pleasure they require to get the same kick. This sleep disruption can also set the stage for some of the disorders discussed previously, such as sleep terrors, sleepwalking and sleep paralysis.

A little while ago I got to work on a project focusing on this interesting topic. This work was led by a super-smart chum from my PhD days, Dr Mike Parsons, now a research scientist at a pharmaceutical company. With a number of others, we worked on data collected from participants of the *Dunedin Multidisciplinary Study of Health and Development* in New Zealand (discussed in Chapter 5). In particular, we wanted to know more about social jetlag in relation to body weight and metabolic dysfunction. There is a difference between being overweight and pretty healthy, and being overweight and having signs of metabolic disorders (such as a large waist, high blood pressure and not a lot of 'good cholesterol').

Parsons chose this topic because it was already known that anything that disrupts our circadian rhythms has the potential to disrupt the balance of energy in our bodies. Earlier research showed that disrupting the circadian rhythm of mice by changing their dark/light cycles resulted in increased weight as well as increased levels of hormones linked to hunger and metabolism, namely leptin and insulin.[46] This animal work was published in the prestigious scientific journal *P-NAS* – to which academics appear to be able to refer without even a flicker of a smile.

In our study, we looked at social jetlag in over 800 people.[47] While we focused on adults (aged 38), social jetlag commonly occurs in adolescence – which is why it is discussed here. We made sure that none of the people we looked at were shift workers, as we were interested in looking at the type of social jetlag that is more commonly found outside of this.

Social jetlag was defined as the difference in the mid-point of sleep between days on which people were free to set their own schedules and days on which they had to work. So, for example, if someone kips from midnight to noon at weekends (their mid-sleep point being 6 a.m.), and 9 p.m. to 5 a.m. on their work days (mid-sleep point 1 a.m.), their social jetlag would be five hours (the difference between 1 a.m. and 6 a.m.).

As expected, we found that greater social jetlag assessed over the past month was linked to both obesity and metabolic dysfunction. Over and above, when we compared obese participants who were metabolically healthy with those who were not, we found social jetlag to be more pronounced in the latter group. The media picked up this story and proclaimed that our weekend lie-in is bad for us.[48] So, does this mean that adolescents should keep their sleep schedule consistent, even if it involves sleep deprivation and misery? I think not. It is the workday schedules that are causing all the drama, and perhaps the weekend lie-in is actually helping our bodies to recover.[49,*] Given what we know to date, thinking hard about what can be done to reduce social jetlag (including considering delaying school times for adolescents, flexible working hours for adults and even daylight-saving time) has the potential for huge public health implications.

What to do?

It appears that the unkind stereotype of adolescents sleeping until noon and partying all night is in part based in biology. We all know that groggy feeling following being woken up before we are ready – our body is not yet prepared to function in the world around us. This is unsurprising as our body is such a finely tuned instrument and we are in quite a different biological state when asleep compared to when we are not. When we wake up in the morning our temperature rises and the level of our stress hormone, cortisol, increases – and these are both under circadian control. Such things help our bodies cope with the day ahead. When we get up earlier than we would like, our body is hollering at us, telling us that we should be asleep. Is this really the best time to force our youths to get out of bed, catch a bus and take an exam?

Scientists have for a long time understood the misalignment between adolescents' biological and social

---

* Some experts recommend that on weekends we allow ourselves to awaken up to two hours later than during the week. This can help our bodies recover from sleep deprivation, while also limiting social jetlag.

timing, and there have been numerous calls over the years to persuade school districts and administrators to start school later in the day. Such changes would put school times in line with biological timing.* After all, sleep is important for learning, memory, emotional regulation and so many other processes that could support good academic and behavioural outcomes at school.

An early project called the Z's to A's Act was discussed in a report that was presented to the US Congress in 1999. Schools that started their days before 9 a.m. were to be offered a grant of up to $25,000 in order to help facilitate a change to start their school days after 9 a.m. The aim of the project was to help encourage schools to start later, resulting in more Zs, which could translate into more A grades. Sadly this bill was not enacted, although other initiatives of this type have made greater progress.

Actually, there was a lot going on before this bill was presented. In 1997 the Minneapolis Public School District declared that children should no longer start their school day at 7.15 a.m., so pushed back the start times for high schools to 8.40 a.m. This change affected thousands of children throughout the district. It was a smart and courageous move. Just think of the potential fallout when changing the timings of a school day. It's been noted that postponing the children's school day by 85 minutes is likely to have an impact on the parents' and carers' own working days. They would have to start their own jobs later in the day or arrange for extra childcare. Or they might risk leaving their teenager asleep, trusting them to get up on time. At the other end of the day, clubs would have to be rescheduled and mealtimes changed. Aside from family chaos, others would be affected too, with teachers needing to figure out what to do with their own children, the crossing guard needing to stop evening traffic in the dark and the transport system seeing a shift in its usage. The controversy surrounding such a decision has not gone

---

* There is an obvious analogy with the incredible work by the celebrity chef Jamie Oliver at transforming school dinners in the UK.

unnoticed. A researcher involved in understanding the consequences of this brave decision in Minneapolis pointed out that since this initial study, school board members in favour of adopting a similar policy have lost their jobs following disapproval from others.[50] People don't like change.

On a more positive note, it was found that the shift did the expected good. Analysing data from the Minneapolis change four years on, it was found that children who had postponed their start times, as compared with those who had not, were more likely to attend school.[51] They also reported feeling less depressed and were less likely to nod off in class. There has been a dragging concern that delaying the start of the school day would lead to later bedtimes for the children, with associated problems. This was not found to be the case and it was discovered that the children who had a delayed school start got more kip than others – in fact, a whopping five hours more sleep per week as compared with the children in other schools. Everyone was a winner, with many teachers and parents reporting sunnier, calmer children who were easier to teach or live with.

This was great news, but perhaps the strongest support of all for shifting school start time comes from a study finding that car crashes among teenage drivers decreased after school start times were pushed back.[52] Decisions about school start times could literally be the difference between life and death. More recently, a systematic review of the literature concluded that the evidence to date supports policy decisions to delay the school day in order to allow for better sleep, and notes that this may well be one answer to resolving the problem of sleep deprivation during the teenage years.[53] There's still more to learn and the authors of the review cautioned that we need further rigorous studies on this important issue.

Starting school at 8.30 a.m. or later (which is pretty standard in the UK but unfortunately less so in the USA) may have economic benefits too, according to a report published by RAND in 2017.[54] It was pointed out that costs might increase initially, with a need to provide night-time lights on sports pitches, for example. However, over the course of a decade, the US economy could benefit by as much as $83 billion brought about by reduced accidents and improved school performance due to extra sleep.

Shifting school start times may help our adolescents navigate their complex worlds. But what if you are reading this as an adolescent who has to get up at the crack of dawn, or a parent of such an adolescent? Is there anything that you can do to improve things? Importantly, there do appear to be a few things that might be useful. First of all, you could set a bedtime. Families seem to give up on this habit over the years, respecting their child's autonomy as they become older. But perhaps that is not such a good approach. One study found that adolescents whose parents set a bedtime during the week went to bed earlier, slept for a longer period and were less sleepy during the day.[55]

Second, it might be a good idea to make bedtime an early one. This was investigated in a study of over 15,000 adolescents. It was found that, as compared with those whose parents imposed a bedtime of 10 p.m. or earlier, adolescents whose parents let them go to bed after midnight were more likely to experience depression and, alarmingly, suicidal thoughts.[56] These associations appeared to be influenced by the amount of time an adolescent spent asleep, as those with a late bedtime got less sleep. While one explanation is that an early bedtime reduces depression, there are others. For example, given associations between evening preference and depression, it is quite possible that adolescents with depression struggle to go to bed early – making it more difficult for their parents to implement this particular routine.

It's been argued that suggesting an early bedtime might fly in the face of biological explanations for changes in sleep timing during adolescence. It's true that you can't just put an adolescent to bed early and expect them to fall asleep without problems. However, a gradual advancement of bedtime can have benefits for sleep and associated areas of functioning.[57] This might be just one of many helpful and protective factors. Overall, an early curfew might do more than just keep adolescents safe at night — it might allow them to get the shut-eye that they need.

Other tips are common to those at other stages of life and include encouraging a consistent sleep–wake routine, avoiding caffeine and removing technology from the bedroom. These and additional tips are discussed in greater detail in Chapter 9.

What else is going on with adolescent sleep?

The bulk of this chapter has emphasised the shift in sleep timing that occurs in adolescence, but that is not the end of the story. There are lots of other things going on with teenagers' sleep. The rich array of sleep disorders mentioned in Chapter 3 (together with many more things that can go wrong with our sleep) remain relevant.

Some of these may take a slightly different form from those seen in children. Take insomnia, for example. In little ones, insomnia may involve a refusal to go to sleep or to sleep alone, but adolescent insomnia may be more similar to what is seen in adults. It might involve long miserable periods of lying in bed unable to sleep. In fact, around one in five adolescents report staying in bed for more than half an hour before they are able to fall asleep.[58] When this happens, just as with adults, treatments that focus on thoughts and behaviours such as cognitive behavioural therapy and mindfulness can be useful.[59]

Then there are changes in the type of sleep experienced. Going back to think about the stages of sleep and what is going on in the brain, we know that certain types of brainwaves are more common during the sleep of children than of adolescents. These include 'delta waves', which are among the brainwaves with the lowest frequency and largest amplitude, and 'theta waves' (both of which occur during deep 'slow-wave sleep'). These types of brainwaves have been reported to decline by over 50 per cent across adolescence, and this change is believed to be closely tied to the developing brain.[60] In contrast, adolescents spend longer than children in lighter sleep.[61]

The friendship effect

Much of the work discussed up to this point has involved measurements of physiological variables. However, some of the science focusing on adolescence has involved scientists asking participants about different aspects of their lives, such as how they might feel. But here lies a problem. The sensible answers provided by adolescents keen to impress an important-looking adult may provide only one window into their possibly colourful worlds. Is the average adolescent really going to divulge information about their most secret thoughts and activities to a suit? That is not to say all responses provided by adolescents (or other age groups for that matter) are problematic. However, there is clearly something to be said for considering social desirability, or that some participants may be trying to impress researchers, when looking at responses as well as the social context in which data are collected.

In relation to this, recent studies have taken the sensible step of acknowledging that friends are important in adolescence and inviting them to take part in studies. The importance of peer groups during adolescence is undeniable and some of the most important decisions adolescents make – such as which class subjects to choose, whether to mess around in class or lie to their parents about where they are going, and whether to smoke, drink or do drugs – are done with a friend alongside.[13] Furthermore, videos on social media tell us behaviours that perhaps would never be contemplated alone may be considered entirely appropriate when backed up by friends. A large proportion of adolescence is spent with peers, and intriguingly it seems that during adolescence sleep behaviours can even 'spread' among social networks[62],* – as if a nasty rumour or an unpleasant virus. It seems that peers need to be considered in the research mix if we want the whole picture of how adolescents sleep and function when deprived of it.

---

* In this study, drug use also showed 'spread' and there was a relationship between sleep and drugs, so that when someone reported short sleep their friends were more likely to report using drugs.

A recent study of this type has been conducted by researchers at the University of Pittsburgh. The work was a collaboration between Drs Dana McMakin and Peter Franzen as well as others. In their study, they wanted to know about the effect of sleep length on adolescents' feelings and emotions.[63] The research team took the unusual step of inviting adolescents into the sleep laboratory with some of their friends. They came for a two-night visit to the lab on two occasions, about a week apart. On one of the visits, their sleep was restricted and they were only allowed six hours in bed for one night and then just two hours of sleep the following night. During the other visit, their sleep was extended (they were allowed 10 hours in bed for two consecutive nights). In the afternoon of the second day the researchers asked the pairs of friends to discuss a previous disagreement. When adolescents had restricted sleep, they showed more negative emotions (e.g. upset, conflict, withdrawal) during this discussion than when they had long sleep. However, interestingly there wasn't a difference across the two sleep conditions for positive emotions. Other results obtained by the same research team also supported these findings, and when I discussed the results with Dr Franzen he told me: 'In this same study, across two independent samples, when youth were sleep restricted, they had greater physiological reactions to negative auditory sounds, as well as more negative emotional behaviours when discussing a conflict with friends. Together, these results suggest that getting enough sleep is critically important in regulating emotions. Emotions tend to run both high and low during adolescence, and getting too little sleep may make this worse. This may be part of the reason that sleep and circadian rhythm disturbances increase the risk for problems like substance use, risk-taking, depression and suicidality.'

Adolescence: a key juncture

There is no doubt that adolescence often involves the pinnacles of emotion. The same passion and rage doesn't usually exist in the same way as we age. Temperate adults may only vaguely resemble the people they once were as adolescents. As to what is going on, adolescence has been described as a time that brains develop to have 'Ferrari engines with Fiat brakes'.[13,64] Scientists have explained the 'Ferrari engines' as being the development of the systems of the brain involved in reward processing and emotions, and that perhaps let us run a little wild. The 'Fiat brakes' refer to the relatively slower development of cognitive control systems in the prefrontal cortex, involved in decision-making and planning, and in keeping us sensible. In reality this is overly simplistic and not all adolescents' brains behave in this way. But what a time of opportunities and risks. Experiences during adolescence really can differentiate life courses, both good and bad.

Thinking back to the early 1990s, I feel less guilty about my inability to rise from my bed and asking my mum to trudge the street with a heavy bag of newspapers. My biology made me do it! I was going to bed later and my internal day was possibly longer than ever before. The light around me might not have played the desired role in helping me go to sleep and wake early too. My social life was blossoming and I wanted to do well in my exams. Yet, I was trying to get up earlier than ever before. It was a collaborative effort, but I am pleased to say that together we ended up earning enough money to purchase that hi-fi system from that electronics store. It lived in my bedroom and provided copious amounts of pleasure – although I'm not sure it ever did much for my sleep.

CHAPTER FIVE

Sleep in Youth: Sleep, Atypical Development and Mental Health

Schoolchildren (6–12 years) recommended 9–12 hours of sleep per 24 hours
Teenagers (13–18 years) recommended 8–10 hours of sleep per 24 hours[1]

On the evening of 17 January 2015, my husband and I were flopped on the sofa watching a box set. I never really watch TV for more than five-minute bursts without succumbing to the urge to check my email. That evening an email grabbed my attention entitled 'Your research!' It was from Debbie from North America who was aware of my scientific papers drawing links between sleep, behavioural and emotional problems, and who wanted to share her story with me. Her son, Ben, aged just 10, had displayed some alarming behaviour. He attacked other children and constantly had suicidal thoughts. His schoolwork was poor and his attitude worse. He hated everyone and everything. Ben's teachers had reached a breaking point and his school was threatening to exclude him. His family were desperate to understand what was going on, so Debbie pushed for a number of consultations. He was eventually diagnosed with oppositional defiant disorder (ODD). That could have been the end of the story, but upon having Ben assessed in a sleep laboratory something unexpected was discovered. There were curious pauses in his breathing while he was asleep, leading to decreased oxygen in his blood. Desperate for oxygen, he would wake up with a start. He was found to have sleep-disordered breathing (mentioned in Chapter 3), which was resulting in extremely disturbed sleep. To imagine how disruptive this disorder can be, experts sometimes draw an analogy with being poked in the arm every few seconds

during the night.[2] We would not be able to get the deep and
peaceful sleep that we need to behave in a regulated way, to
feel happy and to learn effectively. After various procedures
aimed at reducing his sleep-disordered breathing, such as
removing his adenoids and tonsils,[*] Ben's sleep improved –
and so did the problems with his behaviour and emotional
regulation. His performance at school picked up too. Debbie
is now on a mission to spread the word, feeling it was somewhat
by chance that she stumbled upon the correct diagnosis that
had eluded his paediatrician, counsellors, psychologists, family
and school mediators for so long. She thinks that sleep should
routinely be assessed to make sure that problems of the type
experienced by Ben are not driving behavioural or learning
difficulties the child might be experiencing. Debbie is keen to
promote knowledge among parents, teachers and healthcare
providers about the important role of sleep in childhood and
the dramatic consequences of it going wrong.

Beyond doubt, sleep is important for many things. There
are few areas of our waking life that are not influenced by
it – and, in an endless spiral, these same areas of life can also
affect the way that we sleep. It's no wonder that Ben was
struggling with so many aspects of his life when his sleep was
being so cruelly disrupted. Children need to get good sleep
to function well. But as well as causing problems, sometimes
poor sleep can be the consequence of mental health and
behavioural difficulties.

Mental health problems are extremely common, affecting a
huge proportion of us.[3] Ask a group of teenagers about the
way they think and behave, and perhaps a quarter will divulge
information to suggest that they have already experienced a
mental health disorder that has caused a big problem for their
lives.[4] And these are related to sleep.[5]

Even the lucky few who sail through life avoiding severe
mental anguish will have some difficulties. It is now clear that

---

[*] Not every child who snores or has sleep apnoea needs surgery. This
is decided on a case-by-case basis by medical experts.

most problems of this type exist on a continuum, meaning that we all have at least some of the symptoms of various mental health disorders. After all, who can say they have never felt at least a little bit anxious or depressed? This chapter is relevant to us all.

Sleep in children with disorders of brain development

A good place to start when considering mental health disorders is the *Diagnostic and Statistical Manual of Mental Disorders*, which is currently in its fifth edition (DSM-5).[6] This book classifies different mental health problems and is sometimes used as the basis for clinicians to diagnose problems. When we talk to our doctors about mental health problems, they could well be pondering the contents of this book.

One category listed within the DSM-5 is neuro-developmental disorders. These include a wide range of problems including intellectual disabilities, autism spectrum disorder, ADHD and Tourette's syndrome. These disorders can have a profound impact and some are common. Go into your average classroom and it's likely that one or more children will be suffering from ADHD,[7] for example.

Raising a child with certain disabilities can at times bring challenges. Occasionally, there are endless hospital appointments, and arranging babysitting for a child with difficulties can bring extra considerations. Sometimes this makes it incredibly challenging to continue with employment or engage in social events. Parents can feel they are unable to go off duty – day or night. In researching this book, I spoke to Mitch, father of six-year-old Charlie who has been diagnosed with global developmental delay with an auditory processing disorder and some autistic traits. He described Charlie as needing less sleep than the other members of the family, going to bed later and getting up earlier. He talked me through Charlie's night wakings too: 'Charlie will, every now and then, wake at around 2 a.m., and stay awake for any time between one and six hours. He sometimes lies quietly in bed, if one of us lies with him, but other times he will be up. When that happens, he's pulling books off of the shelves or clothes out of cupboards or climbing on windowsills. This means that we need to supervise him and can't doze off ourselves. So on those nights, we have a disrupted night's sleep, and sometimes a complete lack of it. And Charlie doesn't seem to need to 'catch up' on sleep after a night like that, so there's not a chance for us to catch up, either.' Going on to talk in more detail about the effect that Charlie's sleep has on the other family members, Mitch continues: 'We have a very short amount of child-free time each day. If Charlie is up until 9 p.m., and we want to go to bed at 10 p.m., that gives us just an hour of child-free time. Or we snatch a bit more child-free time and go to bed later instead, which makes us sleep deprived and tired. Neither option is great. Our other children are affected, too ... Charlie is always awake when our other children are, so there's no time for me to do one-on-one listening to my older daughter's reading in the evening, for example.' Mitch goes on to talk about the challenges of being away from his son. 'We can't really leave Charlie for the night either. It's a big ask to get someone to look after a child who may be up for hours in the night. We can probably – just about – handle the lack of sleep, disrupted nights, and lack of child-free time at the moment. But when we are 50, or 60, or 70? Charlie has a life-long disability so this is a life-long problem for us, and one we do worry about.'

When I share this story with Nisha, an expert on neurodevelopmental disorders who has a son who has been diagnosed with ADHD, she is entirely unsurprised and tells me that she hears this sort of story all the time from her clients. This type of experience perhaps provides a new perspective to the frustrating 30 minutes of night waking that so many other parents experience when their children are young. It also emphasises that support needs to be available for parents of children with neurodevelopmental disorders to allow them to rejuvenate following missed sleep.

Despite the issues that Mitch is dealing with, he is also positive and points out that while the term disability is sometimes used to refer to impairment or disadvantage, we should not forget that people are so much more than the difficulties they experience. 'Parenting a child with a learning disability certainly brings its challenges, but the joy that Charlie brings outweighs those a hundred times over.' He even tells me about advantages associated with Charlie's disturbed sleep. 'If we ever need him to stay up late at a wedding, or on a flight, he can be relied on to do so with good humour and energy. The energy and enthusiasm he has during all the many hours he is awake – during the day and night – is a fundamental part of his character, and one I admire and adore. Charlie loves life.'

What is going on with the sleep of children with disorders of brain development depends very much on their specific disorder. Take Down's syndrome, for example. Certain physiological features associated with this disorder, such as low muscle tone in the throat, can result in difficulties breathing during the night. This makes sleep-disordered breathing common in those with this syndrome[8] and can lead to a concerning disruption to sleep.

Other disorders of brain development may be associated with sleep in entirely different ways. Autism spectrum disorder (ASD) is a disorder of brain development that at its core involves problems with social interactions, communication and repetitive behaviours and interests. Children with ASD can find it particularly hard to fall asleep and to stay asleep. They may also sleep less than others.[9] It's not entirely clear why this is. However, overall these sleep patterns reflect a child developing in an unusual way. One intriguing possibility is that unusually low levels of the darkness hormone melatonin is released by some of those with ASD or that their melatonin circadian rhythm is abnormal.[10] This could mean that children with this disorder are missing out on an important physiological cue to go to sleep.

But there are other explanations too. Just think about what it involves to be diagnosed with ASD.[6] While of course no two children with this disorder are the same, characteristic symptoms may interfere with sleep.[2] Among other things, those diagnosed can be very sensitive to certain stimuli, such as noise. Some children with ASD clasp their hands firmly over their ears, trying to block out the sounds around them that have become overwhelming. The midnight screams of foxes or aeroplanes rumbling overhead may do little to disturb the sleep of most people but may make nodding off impossible for those who are particularly sensitive to sounds. Whereas clocks tick unnoticed in countless bedrooms, each stroke may reverberate in the head of someone who is sensitive to noise, stopping them from sleeping. As routine, sleep experts advise people to keep the environment 'just so' in order to sleep well. We should reduce noise and optimise temperature, for example. Where this is not possible, and there are loud noises outside or the night is particularly hot, this may disrupt sleep to the greatest extent in those who are most sensitive to these things.

Then there can be an insistence on things staying the same. A child with ASD could need to get dressed in a certain order every day, always starting with their socks. Or perhaps, that child might need to cross the road at the identical place on the way to school each day, at the second set of traffic lights. It's not unthinkable that someone with this disorder could also like their bedroom to be 'just so' before drifting off. Perhaps teddy bears should be lined up in a certain order, with the little ones clustered in the centre or arranged by the colour of their fur. There may also be a preference for the blind to sit at a certain height in the window frame, letting in precisely 1cm of light. Parents may struggle to recreate this scene unerringly, and subsequent stress and inability to sleep could prevail.

But we shouldn't always assume that the disorder is at the root of the sleep problem. Those with disorders of brain development may also experience a range of other sleep problems that are unrelated to their disorder. Perhaps refusal to sleep alone is not always due to a diagnosis but is a result of not having learned to fall asleep without parental involvement, just as with so many other children.

When restless nights follow restless days

Other reasons that disorders of brain development and sleep difficulties so often pair up are highlighted when considering ADHD. This is a disorder that typically begins in childhood and is characterised by inattention and/or hyperactivity. Although symptoms differ from one person to the next, someone with ADHD might struggle to pay attention during class, or may make endless mistakes in their work. Even when spoken to directly, they may fail to respond, appearing to be somewhere else mentally. It can be almost impossible to sit still and a child with this disorder might squirm in their seat or get up when it is inappropriate to do so. They might talk endlessly, interrupting conversations and finishing sentences for others. And then there are sleep problems – restless nights may follow restless days.

Yes, children with ADHD can be sleepless, but there can be other sleep disorders too. They may be more likely to experience sleep apnoea, where breathing stops for an alarming number of seconds during sleep. Periodic limb movement disorder is also common.[5] This disorder involves repetitive and stereotypical limb movements, such as an extension of the big toe, which could be accompanied by bent joints of the ankle, knee, hip or even the upper limbs. As this all occurs when we are resting, it can result in impaired sleep. Intuitively, one might expect that features of ADHD would result in poor sleep, as feeling 'on the go' is unlikely to be conducive to restful shut-eye.

But there are other explanations too. Missing out on slumber and experiencing exhaustion may be expressed by displays of increased energy and excitability and resemble ADHD symptoms in children.[11] Such findings have even led some to ask whether in some cases, behaviour that appears to be symptomatic of ADHD might in fact reflect a sleep disorder.[12] Yet doctors often ignore the possibility that sleep problems are leading to hyperactivity. Nisha, the expert in neurodevelopmental disorders, tells me that her own child was diagnosed with ADHD at the age of five and prior to that nobody had ever asked about his sleep. She considers this to be a big issue, as resolving a sleep problem in a child can have incredibly positive knock-on effects on their behaviour and concentration during the day. The literature backs this up, and removing tonsils to allow children to breathe well at night, or something as simple and non-invasive as fixing a bedtime routine can sometimes help.*

The ADHD–sleep puzzle involves the added dimension that the drugs used to treat ADHD symptoms can sometimes disrupt sleep. Some children are given stimulants to help them cope with their symptoms. This may sound like an unlikely treatment, however the idea is that the brain of someone with ADHD may not be producing enough of the neurotransmitter dopamine.† This treatment increases it to an optimal level, and brain areas involved in attention and in being able to control behaviour are effectively given a boost. A common side-effect of these drugs, however, is to have problems sleeping. This may either be because the stimulant is still active in the body, preventing sleep, or because the drug is wearing off, resulting in a return of ADHD symptoms just as a child is preparing to hit the hay. This certainly reflects Nisha's own experiences. She tells me: 'Before my son started on methylphenidate, he had no sleep problems. Although this drug has been hugely effective in aiding his attention and focus, we have all had to endure the side-effect of the lack of sleep. If we are lucky, on a school night he will fall asleep naturally at about 1 a.m. As a child who normally likes his sleep, and functions well on between 10 and 11 hours, for him to then have to be up at 7 a.m. for school makes it really hard. We have tried good sleep hygiene, it just doesn't work when he's taken his medication. The only way around this is to give him melatonin, which I have a huge problem with as it has not been tested on children.'

---

* This is not to imply that all ADHD-like behaviour is due to sleep problems.
† Dopamine is involved in a variety of different processes including feelings of pleasure and pain.

Nisha suggests I talk to some of the parents who have children with ADHD and with whom she works. She reaches out to them and three respond. Their stories differ from Nisha's – but are all similar to one another. All three describe a situation where their child suffered terribly from sleeplessness from a very early age. One describes a night nanny 'admitting defeat' after a week spent at their home. Another describes trying to settle her child to sleep 27 times in a single night. All three describe the relief at having discovered melatonin, which they have all found to be effective in resolving their problems.* This might be because children with ADHD with difficulties falling asleep are often night owls, with a later melatonin onset as compared with other children,[14] so taking this drug before bedtime can let their bodies know that it's time to sleep. But this is not the end of the story, and problems can remain. For example, one parent mentions melatonin wearing off and her child waking in the middle of the night. Another explains how her child has started questioning his diagnosis and refusing to take melatonin now that he is a teenager. She tells me: 'I was once woken at 4 a.m. by the front door slamming. My son had left me a note saying he was going out to kick a ball about – but luckily he came back once I called him. He is now refusing to go to school, which is partly down to tiredness, as he often doesn't get off to sleep until 5 a.m. If there was one thing I could rectify as part of his ADHD it would be his sleep.'

There are other explanations about why children with ADHD may experience sleep problems and one possibility is that some of these children are experiencing depression, which is driving the association. After all, the links between sleep and depression have been described as amongst the most robust within the field of psychiatry. It's even the case that disturbed sleep can be used as a feature to diagnose depression.[6]

---

* A recent review pointed out that further evidence is needed to confirm the efficacy, optimal dose range and other issues associated with melatonin use (as well as other drugs) to address sleep problems in those diagnosed with ADHD.[13]

Given that depression might be important in explaining why people with ADHD (and a whole range of other difficulties for that matter) suffer from problems nodding off, what do we know about sleep and depression?

Feeling blue and can't sleep

It can be difficult to think of a child experiencing depression as it seems so much at odds with what childhood often is. Good times and fun can be accompanied by boundless enthusiasm and wonderment in the world. But throw in friction with a friend at school, or a missed penalty at football practice, and a child's light can dim. Throw in some of the cruellest things that life has to offer, the death of a loved one, a messy divorce between parents or bullying and social rejection, and it's unsurprising that some children can go on to develop depression.

It's not that such events bring about depression in all children. Some forge forward with few ill effects, but others may struggle. Some children have a genetic vulnerability for developing emotional difficulties, which is only triggered when they come face to face with problems in the world. Bruce Ellis, a professor of family studies from the University of Arizona, sometimes refers to a Swedish proverb about 'orchid' and 'dandelion' children.[15] There are orchid children who are extremely sensitive to the environment, whether good or bad. Stressful life experiences can trigger them to become ill, but they might also respond exceptionally well to therapies aimed at supporting them. Anyone who has owned an orchid will relate to this. Get it right and we have the most beautiful plant to admire, but get it wrong and the plant will not be able to flourish. Then there are the dandelion children whose armour seems impenetrable and will thrive no matter what the circumstances. Hardy dandelions flourish in any old environment, providing children with hours of fun and gardeners just as much frustration.

Sadness and irritability are central features of depression. Other symptoms include lack of interest or enjoyment in the world around us, change in our appetite or weight, and feeling quite worthless. Among these key symptoms are problems with our sleep. If we suffer from insomnia or hypersomnia (excessive sleepiness) nearly every day, we would get a tick in a box and move that bit closer to receiving a diagnosis.

Unsurprisingly then, when we talk to children experiencing depression many report they have problems sleeping. This can take different forms and some will even tell us they sleep too much. I discuss this with a collaborator, Professor Erika Forbes, based at the University of Pittsburgh, who shares my interest in the links between children's sleep and emotional problems. She tells me: 'I've heard people with hypersomnia say that sleep is so rewarding and waking life is so difficult that they only feel good when they are sleeping.' However, too much sleep is not the usual pattern and one problem that is reported time and time again is insomnia. Children with depression are also struggling to sleep at night. So far, this seems pretty straightforward, but delve deeper and things get confusing. While depressed children tell us they are not able to sleep, when we wire them up and investigate their sleep in a laboratory, it's sometimes hard to see these sleep problems. In other words, depressed children are saying that they sleep poorly, but the physiological evidence from polysomnography (the technique used to monitor sleep described in Chapter 1) does not always support this.[16]

This is particularly interesting as when we look at adults diagnosed with depression we don't typically find this gulf. Rather, adults with depression often say they don't sleep well, which can be corroborated in the sleep lab. In fact, some of these unusual sleep patterns revealed in the laboratory are so common in adults with depression that they are even considered to constitute some kind of biological evidence that someone actually has depression. An overwhelming tendency towards REM sums up some of the key changes nicely. After those with depression have fallen asleep, REM sleep often arrives unusually quickly. Those with depression are also more likely to spend a greater proportion of their sleep in REM and the frequency of rapid eye movements within REM is also increased. Unsurprisingly, this means that deeper sleep has to take a bit of a back seat.

So, what might be going on in the children who say they can't sleep but appear to sleep perfectly normally when assessed in a laboratory? Perhaps they don't really have sleep problems after all? Could children experiencing depression need sleep so badly that their bodies manage to steal it? Instead, the discrepancy between what is said and shown is perhaps due to the depression making children feel that everything is bad (including their sleep). Another possible explanation is that the techniques we use to measure sleep are not currently sensitive enough to register the problems that are occurring.

As well as depression leading to sleep problems, sleep problems might also cause depression. Experts in this field consider this particularly likely. Just think about how someone feels after a night of poor sleep. We may feel tired and be less likely to go out and enjoy ourselves. Perhaps we will cancel an exercise class or a date with a friend after a night of sleeplessness. We're pulling out of the very positive life events that might be helping to keep depression at bay.[17]

Other explanations as to why insomnia and depression are bedfellows include them being part of the same genetic cluster. This means that these disorders may be inherited together. We are born with a vulnerability to both depression and disturbed sleep, a conclusion that has been reached from my own research[18] as well as that of others.[19]

Different explanations focus on the sleep-deprived brain, which may be behaving in an atypical way and increase vulnerability to depression. One brain area that could be affected after a night of poor sleep is the amygdala. This is an almond-shaped structure located deep in the brain. It is believed to play a key role in our emotions and in the levels of anxiety that we experience. One study found that, when participants were deprived of sleep for around 35 hours their amygdala showed a greater response to emotionally negative pictures compared with those who had not been sleep deprived.[20] Not getting enough sleep had caused a greater emotional response by the brain. What is more, participants also appeared to be less able to control their emotions – as shown by weaker links between the amygdala and parts of the brain regulating this area.

Other theories explaining the sleep–depression link focus on the immune system. Studies have found that when we disturb sleep we experience inflammation in our bodies as if we are fighting an infection or healing from an injury.[21] In other words, if you take blood from people who are sleep deprived you might see high levels of inflammatory markers such as C reactive protein, which can be useful in fighting infections. Could this help to explain why those who are at risk of or experiencing depression also show high levels of inflammation?[22] This could explain more than just the sleep–depression links, as it is now known that inflammation is linked to a whole host of psychopathologies.[23]

Sleep and suicide

Suicide is a deeply concerning issue associated with depression, and one which also links up with sleep. If we look at a group of teenagers with depression, those reporting lots of sleep problems may also be more likely to think about death and suicide compared with those with no sleep disturbances or minor ones.[24] Attempting to unravel the sleep–suicide link, a group of researchers from Manchester and Oxford universities interviewed 18 adults who had major depressive disorder and had experienced suicidal thoughts or behaviours.[25] The researchers wanted to understand more about how sleep is related to thoughts about or attempts at ending one's life. A few explanations emerged. At night, friends and family are not available to intervene in a crisis, and there is a general lack of other support too, which can increase suicidal behaviour. Missed sleep also makes you feel dreadful, which then makes everyday life more difficult. The final reason was that sleep can provide a temporary relief from it all and missing out on this can be unbearable. Our slumber provides a refuge at the most difficult times of our lives. 'I can't help but wonder if there is a circadian story too,' said Professor Erika Forbes, when we discussed this paper. 'We know that pain intensity, impulsivity and substance use, among other things, fluctuate throughout the day and night. That may also help to explain the sleep–suicide link.'

Nightmares are another aspect of sleep linked to suicide. These ghastly dreams are more common among young people who think about suicide compared with those who don't.[26] There are many ways of explaining this association. One possibility is that distress experienced during the day spills over into the night, just as those suffering from post-traumatic stress disorder (PTSD) may have recurrent distressing dreams about the event or the emotions associated with it. It's perhaps difficult to know what to do with this information. People are experiencing disturbed sleep and nightmares all the time, whereas far fewer are thinking about suicide. Nobody would suggest that just because teenagers are struggling with sleep they are automatically at risk of suicide. However, information about sleep, together with careful consideration of what else is going on in these teenagers' lives could potentially put doctors and others in a stronger position to act quickly and decide when someone is in particular need of help. People who are suicidal may particularly require help at night to be carried safely through their darkest times.

Too scared to sleep

One disorder that commonly occurs with depression is anxiety. Feeling tense, wound up and anxious is never conducive to nodding off. People sometimes report that when their partners go away, they simply don't sleep so well. That is sometimes the case even if said partner is more like Homer Simpson than Dolph Lundgren. It's unclear what these languid partners might do in case of a horribly scary incident. Perhaps dive under the covers? But sometimes just having someone snore next to us allows us to diffuse responsibility, puts us at ease and permits us to fall into a more blissful sleep.

The same is true of children. When they are feeling anxious they also tend to sleep poorly. Around the age of six, when thought processes allow children to start dealing in the abstract and acknowledge the realities of life, nightmares commonly occur, and there may be a peak in children's reluctance to sleep alone. Unlucky family members might become recipients of nightly bed-gatecrashings too.

Thea, the ex-accountant whom we met in Chapter 2, is now in better health and her sons are developing into wholesome and happy children. As with most children, they experience problems from time to time. Thea describes to me difficulties that her eldest son William, aged six, has experienced with anxiety, causing him to have problems sleeping. She mentions one experience where the radio was on and William overheard news about the *Charlie Hebdo* massacre, in which 12 people were killed and 11 injured. She tells me: 'He couldn't get to sleep in the normal way for a few weeks. The worries usually came out just before bed. Lots of questions about guns and Paris and why, why, why?'

When you delve into the literature, the links between child anxiety and sleep problems initially seem clear. One of the key researchers in this area is Professor Candice Alfano, mentioned in Chapter 3. Alfano has spent much of her career working with anxious children. She typically focuses on clinically significant cases, and there is a difference between the worry that many children experience when joining a new school or taking part in show-and-tell, and that which prevents someone leaving the house without immense distress. In one of her reports, she found that alarmingly almost 9 out of 10 of the anxious children in her study were reported by parents or clinicians to have some type of sleep problems – such as difficulty getting to sleep, nightmares or sleeping too much or too little.[27]

My own work has addressed the links between anxiety and sleep in children too. One of the projects on which I collaborated was led by Professor Erika Forbes.[28] Work had already been done that showed children who say they are anxious also say they don't sleep very well. However, Forbes wanted to further understand this link by looking at the way these children slept in the lab. She compared three groups of children and adolescents: those with anxiety disorders, those with major depressive disorder and those with no history of a mental health disorder. When looking at information from the sleep laboratory, the pattern of results was not straightforward. Consistent with some previous work, depressed adolescents did not have many 'objective' sleep differences (or rather those assessed using polysomnography) compared with a healthy control group. However, a few differences emerged for the anxiety group. For example, she found that those with anxiety had less slow-wave (deep) sleep than those in the other groups. The anxious group also woke up more at night compared to those with depression. They seemed to be on red alert. This suggested that not only do anxious children often report differences, but you can also see certain differences in their sleep patterns.

But some researchers think the situation might be more complex than this. Going back to Alfano, her team published a paper in 2016 where they looked at nightmares in anxious children.[29] The team pointed out that most of the previous studies of anxiety and nightmares had focused on parental reports of the latter. She wondered whether the children were also reporting these bad dreams. The team asked the parents if their children had nightmares and they asked the kids themselves too. They found that both the parents and children with anxiety were more likely to report bad dreams compared with those without anxiety. So far the picture seemed pretty clear: anxious children have more nightmares than those who are not anxious. But then the story got murkier. The team tried to get real-time data. Instead of asking parents and children to report something that may have happened in the distant past, they interviewed the children every day for a week about their sleep the night before and in particular their nightmares. The researchers were surprised to find absolutely no differences between the anxious and non-anxious children. When I last spoke to Alfano – after more than a decade of her researching this topic – she seemed pretty convinced that at least some of the robust associations between sleep and anxiety might be to do with the way anxious children report situations. 'We are seeing these types of discrepancies again and again in our data and have come to believe anxious kids simply have low "self sleep-efficacy" – meaning that they just don't think they are good at sleep,' Alfano concludes.

So, what to do about the anxious child who is not sleeping well or believes that they are bad at sleeping? Counter-intuitively, the very behaviours that parents use to support and reassure their children might actually contribute to poor sleep quality and reinforce anxiety.[30] Lying next to children as they fall asleep might be comforting for them, but the big bodies of adults moving about and the noises they make could also reduce their sleep quality. Being there as children fall asleep could also be interpreted as somehow validating their belief that the dark is scary and that bodyguards are necessary to help them get through the night safe and sound. Better techniques include tailoring methods for the anxious child, such as providing a 'bedtime pass' allowing them to get out of bed just once after lights out, which can provide reassurance even if not used.[2]

In the case of Thea's son William, who stalls bedtime when he gets anxious, Thea tells me that she feels she hasn't always approached the situation correctly. She says: 'On one night when he couldn't get to sleep, I made the – on reflection, stupid – mistake of suggesting that he wouldn't be allowed to do the things he wanted to do the next day. I realised very quickly that this only served to heighten his anxiety and make it worse. Once I adjusted my response to being totally chilled and laid back, he started to fall back into a better pattern.'

Missing sleep and feeling psychotic

The links between disturbed sleep, anxiety and depression are among the most well-established within the field of psychiatry. By contrast, far less is made of the association between poor sleep and one of the most severe mental health conditions – schizophrenia. This disorder is misunderstood and seems to be confused with 'Jekyll and Hyde' behaviour, but it's not actually like that. It's a psychotic disorder, which instead of involving a split personality, is characterised by difficulties interpreting reality. It can be difficult to know if something is coming from the inside or the outside of your mind, or where other things end and we begin. Those with schizophrenia may suffer from delusions, holding a belief that stubbornly remains, regardless of evidence to the contrary. Delusions can be quite varied and someone with schizophrenia could believe that the child coughing in the chip shop is sending a hidden message about a forthcoming alien invasion or that the bus driver waiting for them to find their ticket is in love with them. Talking to someone experiencing a psychotic episode confirms just how frightening these experiences can be. Someone may be so frightened that it's easy to believe that their life is in danger. Hallucinations are also very common and involve perceiving something that is simply not there. A voice might instruct someone with schizophrenia to do something. These things do not exist but are so realistic that it can be difficult to believe that. Such disorders can be hugely distressing and debilitating.

Much of the work tapping into this area focuses on adults because psychosis is most likely to occur during this stage of life. It seems that adults with schizophrenia, as compared to those without, may get less sleep, take longer to fall asleep and are more likely to spend time awake during the night.[31] But what about these associations in youth? This has not been looked at to the same extent, but where it has been, it seems that those who revealed problems sleeping and feeling sleepy reported more psychotic-like experiences than those who did not.[32]

Other night-time occurrences may also be linked to psychotic experiences. Nightmares are an obvious thing to look at, given that the hallucinations are sometimes considered to be dream-like in nature. A study investigating this questioned mothers about their children's nightmares when aged between two and a half and nine years of age. Children whose mothers reported frequent problems were, when they reached the age of 12, more likely than others to report such psychotic experiences as hallucinations or delusional beliefs.[33]

So, the way we sleep appears to be related to psychotic experiences, but why? A few years ago I collaborated with researchers from Birkbeck, University of London and the University of Oxford to examine sleep quality and psychotic experiences in a large sample of 16-year-old twins.[34] Our results seemed to suggest that these difficulties co-occur because they are inherited together and also because of environmental experiences. The next piece of the puzzle is to understand the pathways by which genetic and environmental influences impact upon sleep quality and psychotic-like experiences. For example, how do genes and our life experiences influence the developing brain? How might they influence the development of the bilateral thalamus – a part of the brain involved in sleep, which appears to be smaller in adolescents at high risk of psychosis?[35]

Avoiding a rest: missing out on sleep and behaving badly

Those who don't sleep well find it difficult to regulate their emotions.[36] Although this has mainly been used to explain why disturbed sleep can co-occur with anxiety and depression, it also follows that children who haven't been sleeping well might yell, scream and thump the other child annoying them. The lid on their behaviour is loose at best. Research finds this to be true, and there are links between not getting sufficient sleep and behaving badly.[5]

But there is bad behaviour and *bad behaviour* and psychologists have spent many years carving this up in different ways. One theory, which perhaps yields the greatest fascination among the general public, is the idea that certain people who show disruptive behaviours such as aggression and rule breaking could be 'psychopaths'. Although there are adults who can be diagnosed as psychopaths, this is not a label that should be applied to children. However, some children share personality features with adult psychopaths and are at risk of developing psychopathy. They behave in more callous, unemotional and insensitive ways than others. They are primarily concerned with looking after number one, are less responsive to the distress of others and feel little guilt. There is a difference between people who behave badly and feel bad about it and those who behave badly and don't.

My own interest in sleep and psychopathic traits stemmed from when I was a PhD student at King's College London. For a short while I shared an office with a fellow student, Essi Viding, now a professor at University College London. Viding's studies focused on the development of callous and unemotional traits in children. Although she does not comment on individual cases, she described some of the children she studied as charming when things were going the way they wanted, but capable of incredible cruelty if someone was standing in their way. She found it chilling that the children did not seem to feel a shred of empathy for others that they had hurt and viewed everything in terms of whether it was to their advantage.

A lot is known about people with high levels of psychopathic traits and one striking feature of these children is that they are typically not very anxious. If you were able to peer inside their brains, you might see that when they encounter things that cause big emotional reactions in most people (such as a picture of someone feeling very distressed) their brains just wouldn't respond in the same way. The amygdala, a part of the brain involved in emotional responding, remains pretty chilled out at times when it would be going into hyperdrive in other people.[37] But what about their sleep? Over the years, I'd discussed this with Viding time and time again but very little was known, although she seemed pretty confident that the participants she typically recruited into her studies wouldn't be experiencing sleepless nights. This was an interesting hypothesis as pretty much all of the other traits studied in the field of psychopathology, whether autism spectrum disorder, anxiety or schizophrenia, are associated with poorer quality sleep.

Other commitments meant that it took us years to get our acts together to test this hypothesis. Even then, the project only progressed thanks to a group of incredible students who led this work. Among our questions, we wanted to explore further the known links between sleep and antisocial behaviour, and to also see what was going on regarding these callous-unemotional traits.

In order to do this, we looked at data from more than 1,500 young adults about their sleep quality, disruptive behaviours and callous-unemotional traits. Instead of focusing on those with very severe symptoms, we looked at a typical sample from around the UK. It wasn't that we were expecting our participants to have particularly high levels of callous and unemotional traits, but just as we're all on the anxiety spectrum – with some of us experiencing very few and others experiencing many symptoms – the same is true of callous and unemotional traits. This should come as no surprise when we think of friends and colleagues, as some clearly show much more empathy and experience more guilt than others.

In our study we found a link between sleeping poorly and reporting behavioural problems. This has been found before, but it was reassuring to see that we could replicate this finding, showing that our sample was similar to those used by others. By contrast, there was no association between sleep and callous and unemotional traits. Just because someone reported lacking emotion and being somewhat callous did not mean they slept poorly. This fitted well with our initial expectations.

Before publishing this work, we wanted to see whether our findings were a one-off quirk or if they would replicate. The students therefore collected extra data in what we referred to modestly as 'The Ultimate Sleep Study'.[38] The team asked 338 adults lots of questions about various aspects of their lives. As in the previous study, people claiming to have more disruptive behaviours also claimed to sleep more poorly. We then looked to see whether people who reported having more callous-unemotional traits had poorer sleep. This time our results were slightly different. Now we found that after taking other things into consideration that might affect our results – specifically the age and sex of the participants – higher levels of callous-unemotional traits were actually associated with better sleep! We asked a proportion of the sample – 43 people – to wear a watch-like device called an 'actigraph' for a week. This records when people move and can be used to provide another picture of how they have slept. The general idea here is that when we are active and moving about we are probably awake, whereas when we are inactive and still we are more likely to be asleep. The late Professor Avi Sadeh from Tel Aviv, Israel, a dear colleague and a founding father of the actigraphy technique – having been one of the first scientists to show that it provided a valid way of measuring patterns of sleep and wake – kindly visited us in London to teach us how to use the watches and interpret the data. Although Viding had made predictions many years before, we were stunned to see, yet again, that people reporting higher levels of callous-unemotional traits appeared to sleep better than others. When lying in bed they moved about less than others and spent a greater proportion of their time in bed fast asleep. These findings stand in stark contrast to what is typically found with other aspects of psychopathology, and adds another piece to the jigsaw in understanding what is going on with people who report those traits.

The first time I presented this work at a conference, a lady sidled up to me at the end of my talk and declared: 'You know you're really onto something with this sleep and callous-unemotional stuff. My ex-husband always slept like a log and turned out to be a complete psychopath.'*

How do problems unfold over time?

Another question that has always interested me is whether sleep problems might constitute a red flag for other difficulties. Do sleep problems allow us to predict that the sufferers will go on to struggle in certain areas of life? This is a question I have asked throughout my career. In order to address such

---

*While I don't know her husband, she's right and I'll be interested to see whether other teams explore this further, perhaps even looking at this question in relation to participants of other ages.

questions I have used data from the *Dunedin Multidisciplinary Study of Health and Development* (mentioned in Chapter 4).[39] This study was set up back in the day when wearing polyester trousers and platform shoes was *à la mode*. The study was launched in 1972, to be more precise. The investigators recruited into their study the parents of 1,037 babies born in Dunedin, New Zealand. All babies were born between 1 April 1972 and 30 March 1973. Perhaps nobody knew it at the time, but this was to become one of the world's greatest epidemiological studies. Since recruiting these families in the 1970s, these babies (now middle-aged adults) have been followed up over and over again. Those involved appear to be overwhelmingly dedicated to this study, with hardly any of them dropping out over the years. In fact, when the participants were most recently assessed at 38 years of age, 95 per cent of those alive took part in the study. Anyone who has ever conducted a study of this type will find this mind-blowing. Over 1,000 scientific papers and reports have been published from this study, telling the world about how people develop over time in areas as diverse as their mental, oral and sexual health, as well as their brain and cardiovascular functioning.

I feel able to celebrate the Dunedin study without revealing hidden narcissism, as I have had nothing to do with its immense success. Instead, researchers, including professors Avshalom Caspi, Temi Moffitt and Richie Poulton, have spent years obtaining funding and carefully considering each and every detail of the study. They have allowed researchers like me to test hypotheses using their data. They have nabbed countless awards during their careers.

During my PhD studies, I was able to discuss my ideas with Caspi and Moffitt. One of the very first questions I was desperate to ask was whether children who slept poorly might go on to become adults who suffered from anxiety and depression. Previous studies hadn't examined this fully, but from the literature I thought it made sense that this association existed. I looked at parents' responses to questions about how their children slept when they were five, seven and nine years of age. I then looked to see whether these responses were associated with what the children revealed about their own anxiety and depression when they became young adults.

In our analyses we took into consideration how anxious or depressed our participants were as children. After doing so, we found that those whose parents had reported them having persistent sleep problems as children were more likely to become anxious as adults, compared with those who had not experienced sleep problems in childhood.[40] We eagerly looked to see if the same might be true in respect of depression, but unexpectedly found this not to be the case. There have been more studies of this type since we published this work. However, the specificity we found between sleep and anxiety, but not depression, has not been widely replicated – and instead, it seems that sleep disturbances predict both anxiety and depression.[41] Overall, not sleeping well as a child may well be a red flag for problems of this type later in life.

It appears that children who struggle with their sleeping might be a little more likely than others to develop anxiety and depression later on. Further links have been reported too, with children who are poor sleepers, or who don't get enough shut-eye, more likely to develop problems including psychotic symptoms, bipolar spectrum disorders, addictive behaviours and ADHD later in life.[5,*]

Treat one, treat the other

Years of research has shown us that with few exceptions, sleep and mental health go hand in hand. Mental health issues can be signalled by problems with sleep, and sleep disturbances seem to predict and lead to a range of difficulties with mental health. The list of disorders extends well beyond those listed in this chapter, including post-traumatic stress disorder and obsessive compulsive disorder.[5]

---

* That is certainly not to say that all children who have difficulties sleeping go on to develop other problems. Sleep problems are common in children and in many cases are not associated with other difficulties. However, if you are concerned, always talk to a healthcare provider.

Sleep problems can sometimes be an invisible risk too. Just as with other things such as being bullied at school, parents may simply miss the dangers experienced by their children. Fat chance, some readers may be thinking, recalling beloved small ones padding into their bedroom as soon as their brains even sense wakefulness. But consider adolescents – few wedge themselves in between their unsuspecting parents in the middle of the night, so do adults really know how their offspring are sleeping?

What should we do with the information that sleep problems can forecast later problems? Should we panic next time the children stage a sleep mutiny? No. Not at all. It is clear that there are multiple risk factors for different problems. Take depression, for example. Nobody would suggest that everyone who sleeps poorly develops this disorder. Instead, poor sleep is one of the many things that makes depression more likely – as is being female, getting older, experiencing life stress or feeling lonely. We don't spend time worrying about 'the risk' of getting older, as there is little we can do about it. Besides, these 'risks' come with certain advantages. As an older female, I may be more likely than some to develop depression, but less likely to mug somebody, or hold up the local newsagent.

Instead of using this information to worry about sleeplessness, perhaps we can use it to make a difference? In contrast to the risk factors that we can't change, disturbed sleep is a risk factor that can be addressed, as shown by the case of Ben discussed at the beginning of this chapter. Ben, together with his family, struggled greatly as a result of his sleep-disordered breathing and their lives were greatly improved once this was resolved. This is one reason why this line of research is so important.

Studies have also looked to see whether improving sleep might aid mental health problems. Dan Freeman, a professor at the University of Oxford, and his team are relentlessly pushing forward research into the idea that sleep problems may cause psychosis-like experiences. They are looking to see whether improving sleep has positive implications in respect of psychosis-like symptoms.[42] This work has the potential to be important, so I was delighted to receive an email from Freeman's team asking if I'd like to help out with his research. I agreed without hesitation. The team recruited students who were experiencing insomnia. These 3,755 participants were then either given six weeks of online cognitive behavioural therapy for insomnia or were just left to continue their lives as usual.[43] Those who received the CBT-I (cognitive behavioural therapy for insomnia) had more positive outcomes compared with the others in the study. They experienced reduced insomnia, paranoia and hallucinations, as well as other problems such as anxiety and depression. These effects lasted over time.

In stark contrast to this work and somewhat counter-intuitively, another technique that has been found to help people with major depression is sleep deprivation.[44] Stop someone with depression from sleeping and they might feel remarkably chipper.[45] This surprising suggestion was first made hundreds of years ago, with early observations about the bidirectional links between sleep and depression leading the psychiatrist Johann Christian August Heinroth, born in 1773, to ponder whether sleep deprivation might be an effective treatment for 'melancholia', something he might not have actually tried in his own work.[46] While surprisingly effective, this technique is currently of little value as once patients are allowed to sleep again, which has to happen eventually, their depression typically returns pretty quickly. The excitement about this knowledge is that it could be developed to reduce depression for longer periods. We need to understand the mechanisms by which this technique works in order to do this. For example, the benefits could be associated with resetting the body clock. An increased understanding of the neurotransmitters involved might be useful in helping us develop treatments in the future.

Long may this important work continue, as studies of this type have a huge potential to help so many. These types of studies provide hope that knowing more about sleep may be a route by which to improve mental health. As long as we are doing what we can to embrace the night, we shouldn't lose any sleep over the research out there.

CHAPTER SIX

Becoming an Adult: A Sleep a Day Helps Us Work, Rest and Play

Young adults (18–25 years) recommended 7–9 hours of sleep per 24 hours[1],*

A sharp brain can take us far. Young adulthood can be a time when our brains are taxed like never before. We might enter the job market or take exams to get us there. Perhaps we are figuring out how to look after ourselves outside of the security of family, getting into shape and trying to look our best too? We might be learning to drive or be negotiating complex relationships. It can be hard to keep up. Unfortunately, these adult responsibilities are not coupled with a mature brain. Towards the end of our teenage years our brains are still developing and they are not yet at their mature state.[2] They are vulnerable, and sleep remains important. So how does sleep change when adulthood appears?

Sleeping adults

It would be rude to abandon Captain Obvious (our sleep drive) and the (body) Clock so late in the day. With reference

---

* National Sleep Foundation guidelines about the amount of sleep we need are based on a panel of experts considering literature on sleep duration and its effects on health. It is pointed out that in some cases, individual need may fall outside these recommendations (but that it is rare for requirements to differ substantially from these guidelines). In this report there are also guidelines for babies, children and adolescents, but paediatric sleep researchers often focus on the review by Paruthi and colleagues (2016) instead, referenced in earlier chapters of this book.

to our sleep drive, it takes longer than ever before to feel ready to don our pyjamas. In particular, it has been estimated that while it takes adolescents around 12–14 hours of wakefulness to feel sleepy, it takes adults more like 16.[3] Then there is the clock. In previous chapters, such a big deal was made about puberty shifting adolescents' body clocks that it will probably come as no surprise that adulthood is characterised by a shift back towards earlier bedtimes and rise times. The night-time party is over. This sudden change in sleep timing at around 20 years of age is so common that it has even been proposed as biological evidence to signify the 'end of adolescence'.[4]

There are other general changes too and as we get older we might need slightly less sleep. The 8–10 hours of sleep recommended for teenagers decreases to 7–9 hours for adults,[1] allowing them to fulfil the endless responsibilities associated with this stage of life. While a complete sleep cycle typically continues to take around 90 minutes from start to finish, there are changes in what is happening during that hour and a half. For example, there is a slight increase in the proportion of the lightest type of sleep over time, and a decrease in the type of sleep that is sometimes considered the loveliest: the deep slow-wave sleep that can make us feel so rested, and the REM sleep during which we so often dream.[5] Most depressingly, it is clear that sleep quality gets worse as the years rack up: we take longer to fall asleep and irritatingly wake up more often during the night.[5] Adults are left reminiscing about those long, deep slumbers of youth.

Sleep and brain functioning

And how does sleep relate to brain functioning? Thinking back to some of the central functions of sleep, we know that it can help restore the body and brain. Toxins are cleaned from the brain and it is left primed to cope with the day ahead. Sleep can also help with learning and information processing. New connections are formed and unimportant ones lost. Sleep helps us recalibrate our emotions too, allowing us to cope with the stresses of exams and life. So can we sleep our way to being smart?

To some extent, yes. Data have backed up the idea that sleep is important for learning and functioning well. In a study of young adults it was found that those who reported poor sleep quality, not sleeping for long enough or using medication for their sleep, also performed less well on tasks assessing attention.[6] Those participants also experienced more problems with executive function. This refers to a range of mental processes that allow us to function well – by juggling the different tasks that we have to do, for example. Other studies have supported a link between different sleep habits and functioning, with 16- to 19-year-olds who get poorer quality sleep and less of it, and those whose schedule differs most at the weekend compared with week days, obtaining a lower grade point average.[7]

On the flip side, it seems that we can also 'unlearn' during our sleep.[8] In a study by researchers from the USA, participants were given training aimed at undoing social biases held implicitly. The study focused on gender and racial biases. With regards to the former, gender biases may include people thinking that women are better at arts than they are at science. In their training, participants were asked not to respond when they saw a picture of a woman accompanied by an arts-related word (such as 'theatre'). By contrast, they were asked to press a button when they saw a picture of a woman accompanied by a science-related word (such as 'math'). If they responded quickly enough, a specific tone was played. A different tone accompanied trials that focused on reducing racial bias. In the next stage of the study, participants were played the tones they had heard during the initial training and told to categorise information accordingly. For example, when they heard the tone that had accompanied the counter-bias training for gender, they were required to pair a female face with a science-related word. The participants were then given a 90-minute nap, during which time memories of training were reactivated, by playing one of the two tones repeatedly during slow-wave sleep. It was found that there was a reduction of the pre-existing explicit social biases accompanying the specific tone that was played during sleep. This effect was found straight after sleep and also a week later. Sleep appeared to consolidate implicit learning aimed at reducing undesirable biases.

So sleep appears to be important for learning and unlearning. Missing out on our kip can impair our performance, but how significant are these influences? There have been attempts to quantify the decrease in performance associated with sleep deprivation. How impaired exactly are we when we don't get the sleep that we need? The authors of a meta-analysis conducted in the 1990s concluded that those who are sleep deprived function at the equivalent of only the 9th percentile of those who are not deprived in this way.[9] That should really make us sit up and take note, especially during this stage of life, when performing well can lay the foundations for life ahead.

Although the sleep–performance link is discussed in this section on young adults, the link between sleep and mental performance has also been studied at other stages of life. For example, in children and adolescents, sleepiness, sleep quality and sleep length have all been associated with school performance. Interestingly, in a meta-analysis of these different aspects of sleep, sleepiness showed the strongest link with mental performance.[10] Sleep duration had the weakest. This might be because people differ in the length of sleep needed to function well but might not be getting enough if they feel sleepy. The authors of the report flagged other interesting results too. For example, the associations appeared to be particularly strong in the younger participants – perhaps because sleep is of such great importance at this time of life. In contrast, older children and adolescents are able to last for longer periods without needing to sleep. A role for the prefrontal cortex of the brain (involved in planning and problem solving) was suggested, with sleep deprivation being most significant for the youngest participants who are likely to have a less well-developed prefrontal cortex. The association was also stronger in boys than in girls. This could be because boys develop physically at a slower pace compared with girls – starting puberty later, for example. Dig out some old school photos if in doubt.

So it seems that sleep and mental performance are linked at different stages of life. Could it be that sleep problems during childhood predict the way our brain works later on? This is a question that my colleagues and I have attempted to answer in our own work. Using data from the Dunedin Multidisciplinary Study of Health and Development (described in Chapter 5), we examined the links between sleep and neuropsychological functioning.[11] We considered parents' reports of children's sleep problems and investigated how these were related to brain functioning when the children became teenagers.

We used various tests to tap into the inner workings of different parts of the brain. Mostly, there were no differences, but something fascinating was noticeable. Analysing our data, it became clear that poor sleepers performed worse than others on two specific tests. One of the tests involved drawing a complex picture. Participants were scored for their strategy and accuracy, and this task tapped into their thoughtful planning and visuo-spatial processing.

The second test involved a variation on a dot-to-dot task, including asking participants to connect consecutive numbers and letters. So rather than connecting 1, 2, 3, etc., as you might do in a children's activity book, the participants connected 1, A, 2, B, 3, C, etc. The fact that this latter task stood out was particularly interesting as it put certain demands on working memory and mental flexibility. Performance on this task was likely to reflect the functioning of the prefrontal cortex of the brain and those who had experienced sleep problems as a child struggled with this task. We found the results fascinating as research by others has also flagged working memory as an area particularly susceptible to the effects of sleep deprivation.[12]

While it's possible that sleep problems during childhood had caused some kind of difficulties with the adolescents' brains, we were careful not to rush to this conclusion as there were lots of equally valid explanations. For example, it is possible that the children who slept poorly might have experienced subtle difficulties with the way their brains work to begin with, which we hadn't assessed at the time. These difficulties may have simply remained consistent over time. Given the scope for sensationalising our modest finding, it was a relief that it was not reported by the press in that way.

Overall, it seems that sleep, performance and brain function are indeed linked. So perhaps we can sleep our way to being smart after all. Well, even if we can't sleep our way to being smart, perhaps we can sleep our way to looking smart! This was suggested in a report published in 2016. Scientists assessed faces to try to figure out whether certain features made some look more intelligent than others.[13] One thing they focused upon was the extent of eyelid openness. The idea was that when you are tired your eyelids begin to droop. The cartoon stereotype of lids drooping when tired is based on reality. This state is known to be linked with how alert or tired someone is. In a series of experiments, the authors showed (among other things) that the more open the eyelids, the more intelligent someone was perceived to be. One study reported in the paper involved taking photos before and after participants were sleep restricted. This allowed natural variation in eyelid openness. As expected, participants whose eyelids were more widely open (and so were less likely to be sleep deprived) were perceived by others to be more intelligent. It might well be that the first step to becoming, or looking like, an intellectual is to turn in for the night. Following this reasoning, extra kip might allow us to become versions of Lisa Simpson in no time!

Beauty sleep

The well rested not only look smarter, but might look more attractive too. Not that looks matter, as children are repeatedly told, but young adulthood – when romantic relationships are sometimes consolidated – can be a time when looking attractive can feel particularly important. Whether we care about the way we look or not, the research linking physical attractiveness and sleep is intriguing. In a study in a sleep laboratory in Stockholm, participants were photographed either after a night of normal sleep or after a night of sleep deprivation.[14] In a scenario possibly resembling the internet site 'Hot or Not?', a different set of participants were then asked to rate the attractiveness of the person in the photo. Fascinatingly, those who were sleep deprived were rated as less attractive than others (they were also rated as less healthy and more tired). This perhaps confirms that we don't look our best when we are tired. Another study extended this idea by comparing skin ageing in good and poor-quality sleepers.[15] It was found that good sleepers had better skin than poor sleepers. Their skin was considered to be younger and it showed better recovery from exposure to ultraviolet light. It's not just others who consider the well rested attractive either, they are often quite pleased with their own looks too. In the latter study the good sleepers also considered themselves to be more attractive than did the poor sleepers.

So, perhaps when we have a big day planned and want to look our best, we should add 'sleep' to our preening list. But, we should take time to wake up too. Anyone keen on selfies will know that we don't always look great immediately upon waking. Among other things, fluid can pool around the eyes while people lie asleep, making them look puffy. Stand up and the fluid will drain by gravity. Kip, wake and wait. Be camera ready.

Heavy sleep

We might be able to sleep our way to looking good, but how does sleep relate to our body size? Over recent years studies on sleep and bodyweight have received a huge amount of attention from researchers and the media alike. Perhaps part of the fascination is the alluring possibility that we could

sleep ourselves to looking more like Gigi Hadid or Tyson
Ballou. Surely a more appealing route than a low-calorie diet?

It does seem that lots of different features of our sleep, from
whether we snore, to the quality, length and regularity of our
kip, are associated with our body size. Certainly, a heavy
frame can cause some sleep problems. Excess weight and a
thick neck can result in increased risk of sleep apnoea, for
example. However, what is perhaps less intuitive to most
people is that things could also be working the other way
around: the way we sleep could be contributing to our body
size. As one example, short sleepers appear to be at risk of
gaining weight. This is true not only in adulthood, but also
for babies, children and teenagers.[16] So what could be going
on to explain this? A number of hypotheses have been
proposed.[17]

First of all, when we are sleep deprived we might consume
more calories. A recent meta-analysis focusing on adults
supported this idea showing that missing out on sleep can
lead to an increase in food and drink consumption of
385 calories a day.[18] That number of calories won't buy you
my favourite double chocolate bar, but will take you pretty
close. Over the course of a year this can result in substantial
weight gain and add inches to the thighs.

As to why more calories are consumed, this may be due to
the fact that hormones related to hunger (ghrelin) and feeling
full (leptin) are messed with when we don't sleep for long
enough. In particular, ghrelin increases, making us feel
hungry, and leptin decreases, so we are less likely to feel full.
No wonder we want to eat. We might also increase our
calorie consumption because we have more hours awake and
in which to consume calories. Very few of us eat during our
sleep after all (although, admittedly, some do). It's also been
suggested that our sleep-deprived selves may have different
food preferences. We eat more of the wrong stuff. Greasy
snacks purchased from grotty-looking vans are surely only
appealing late at night and when exhausted? Interestingly,
looking at what might be going on in the brain can also help
us to understand why we desire naughty foods. As discussed

before, it seems that when we are tired parts of the brain involved in complex planning (such as the prefrontal cortex) seem to be somewhat sluggish.[19] By contrast, other parts of the brain involved in motivation and reward (such as the amygdala) seem to be in overdrive. It's no wonder that the instant gratification of some greasy fast food makes so much sense late at night.

A second explanation for the link between short sleep and increased weight is that we simply don't use so many calories when we miss out on our kip. This could be because our body temperature is messed up or because we are too tired to get up and go when awake. Many of us will know that feeling of being exhausted and wanting to do nothing more than flop in front of the TV, burning very few calories. Worse still, if this sedentary activity is accompanied by a large bag of crisps or biscuits, it combines different explanations as to why little sleep might make us gain weight – we are increasing our calorie intake yet decreasing our expenditure.

Workout to sleep

Sleeplessness can make us feel tired and less likely to get up and go. But what else have we learnt about the links between our sleep and our activity levels – and indeed our exercise schedule?

Sleep and exercise is considered in this chapter, as it is often in young adulthood that sporting records are smashed. It seems that the sporting careers of many elite athletes die alongside their early adulthood years.[20] At this stage of life we are often at peak fitness – so how do exercise and sleep marry up? It would seem that the two go together rather well and even a gentle jog, yoga session or kick-about in the park can feel like it's doing wonders for our sleep.

Work hard, rest hard

These impressions are largely backed up by information from reviews and meta-analyses.[21] After exercise we can sleep for longer periods and enjoy sounder sleep. Regular exercise can also influence our sleep architecture, allowing us to enjoy more slow-wave sleep, although decreasing REM sleep too.[22,23] Positive effects of exercise on our sleep help to explain why sleep experts recommend that we take time to exercise during the day.

It was once argued that we should avoid exercise close to bedtime, as one of the many marvellous benefits of activity of this type is to increase levels of alertness – and it makes us hot too. These are things that are somewhat at odds with nodding off. However, more recent recommendations don't add this caveat, noting instead that evenings might be the only opportunity for exercise during busy lives and pointing to data that does not support the idea that night-time exercise is problematic for our sleep.[24,25]

As to why regular exercise can help us sleep well, there are likely to be multiple mechanisms that are not yet fully understood.[26] Exercise can have a positive effect on our circadian rhythms and immune functioning, as well as other pathways, resulting in improved sleep. There are also likely to be indirect routes too. For example, exercise can help improve mood, which is useful given what is known about the links between depression and sleep. Exercise can also help keep weight under control and can therefore prevent us from developing disorders resulting from a heavy frame, such as sleep apnoea.

And what about the sleep of the super-duper athletes – such as Mo Farah, Serena Williams and Lionel Messi? The sleep of top athletes must be off-the-scale incredible, right? Actually, wrong. Studies of elite athletes have often revealed they experience worse sleep than the average person.[27,28] It also seems that sleep quality decreases with overtraining.[29] The link between overtraining and poor sleep is so well established that poor sleep is sometimes used as an index that someone has been training too hard. So, what exactly is going on? Well, first of all, the exercise regime of Mo Farah and co. probably differs from that of most of us. If we're talking statistics, the average person might be lucky to clock up 30 minutes of exercise a day, whereas Farah likely spends a substantial proportion of his waking life stretching and running. There might be an intensity difference too – Farah probably doesn't get lapped while jogging around the park for a start! Whereas the way that many of us train gently nudges our bodies towards a pleasant state of sleepiness, the bodies of elite athletes are put under the most incredible strain. Their immune system may be weakened and their muscles exhausted. The levels of stress hormone cortisol in their bodies may be high too.[30] What is more, recent work on mice has suggested that when they run, activity in certain parts of the brain may actually decrease[31] as if they're slipping into autopilot. Could this apply to humans and mean that under certain circumstances, when bedtime arrives, parts of the brain have actually been less active – and have a diminished need for sleep? Even once athletes get to sleep they may wake up needing to pee during the night, as they've probably been drinking a lot both during and after training to stay hydrated.[32]

Let's think about the lifestyle of an elite athlete. Sports people often enter international competitions – and international competitions involve international travel. A lot of time is likely spent jumping time zones, which will make their bodies confused as to whether it's day or night. Jetlag occurs when our internal processes are out of sync with the external world. Our bodies are working as if in another time zone so might be telling us to go to sleep, when sporting officials are shouting at us to get to the starting line. What is more, the clocks in different parts of our bodies lose synchrony. What can be done about this? Living in harmony with the new time zone helps us adjust. It can be useful to make sure we get morning light and evening darkness, for example. It takes our bodies about a day to adjust for each time zone crossed.[33] Just like turning a big ship, this simply can't be hurried, as the circadian system limits the pace at which the master clock in the brain can be shifted by light. As described by the scientists Russell Foster and Leon Kreitzman, the problem of jetlag for sporting performance doesn't stop with humans and needs to be considered when dealing with animals such as racehorses too. Trainers sometimes adjust food and exercise timings prior to departure in an attempt to reduce this problem.[33] Such techniques are likely to reduce difficulties with jetlag, but will probably do little to resolve the horses' issues with the limited legroom on the flights!

Even without jetlag, the timings of certain sporting events mean that an early bedtime is out of the question. Take the Spanish La Liga soccer matches for example. It has been reported that kick-off is sometimes as late as 10 p.m.[34] While such a kick-off time may seem somewhat late, there is some logic in evening sporting events – avoiding the heat of the day, for example. What's more, our physical performance appears to increase throughout the day, along with our circadian-driven increase in body temperature. Our temperature often peaks between about 5 p.m. and 7 p.m., which may explain why sporting records are so often beaten during the evening.[35] But what works for Peter might not work for Paul, and our own personal-best performances are likely to depend in part on our own unique body clocks. Those who function best in the mornings will probably reach their physical peaks before evening types.[36]

Sleeping in an unfamiliar environment can create unique problems – we all know that feeling of a first night away from home where it seems like our brain is half awake all night. Well, it turns out that this isn't far from the truth. Half of our brain stays somewhat alert when we get our head down somewhere new. This is not greatly dissimilar to the sleep of dolphins (discussed in Chapter 1), who take this one step further and sleep one hemisphere at a time. Whereas sleep typically occurs in both hemispheres in humans, a team of researchers ran a series of studies where they compared sleep during the first and second nights spent in a laboratory in a total of 35 healthy young adults.[37] They found that something incredible happened on the first night, but not the second. Part of the left hemisphere of the brain seemed to stay alert during sleep (falling into a lighter sleep compared with the right side). The team of researchers also found that the left hemisphere was more responsive to sounds in the environment. This suggests that perhaps this part of the brain was acting as a nightwatchman in an unfamiliar environment – ensuring safety when we are somewhere new. This might suggest that even when travelling within time zones athletes need at least an extra night in a new environment in order to sleep well and have the opportunity to perform at their very best at a big event.

Finally, there's stress linked to success. There are sleepless nights and anxiety before huge events. Late nights are spent attending press conferences, celebrating or reliving mistakes. Then there is the need to sell a brand – spending time promoting products in exchange for lucrative sponsorships and ensuring enough charity work to sleep easy. Taken together, it's unsurprising that athletes might spend insufficient time in the land of nod.

Rest hard, work hard

It's a problem that these athletes sleep poorly. When we go back to thinking about why sleep is important, it is clear that to provide someone with the optimal chance to perform at their very best, a good kip is essential. Perhaps of particular relevance to sport, we know that the release of growth hormone, which is so helpful in allowing the body to restore itself, peaks during deep sleep. It's also true that there are links between sleep and many other things that can affect sporting performance. These include cognition, pain perception and tolerance, muscle restoration, immune functioning, glucose metabolism, decision-making, mood, recovery and much more.[38] We've all watched photo finishes of races, footballs hitting the crossbar and tennis balls just failing to make it over the net. Perhaps a good night's sleep can give someone the edge.

So, what to do about this unfortunate situation where athletes might be sleeping poorly when they so desperately need to sleep well? How might we improve their sleep in order to improve their performance? Taking a short nap during the day might be effective, although results are somewhat mixed.[39] It makes good sense that simply telling athletes to prioritise sleep, or extend it is helpful.[34,39] But, as

with all of us, time in bed should only be extended if there is
no time spent in bed awake. If athletes simply lie there, wide
awake and humming the national anthem, this can cause
them to develop negative associations with bedtime, which
will do them no favours.

Good sleep hygiene might be important[39] and extra-long
beds make good sense for sky-high ballers. The nutrition
consumed by an elite athlete is a big deal – and recently
attention has been paid to the types of food that may help to
enhance sleep[38] (see Chapter 9). While all of this is important,
we should encourage good sleep without turning it into a big
deal. After all, who can sleep well when they know they
absolutely must? Just as those with insomnia are told that they
will live to fight another day after a bad night of sleep, it
might be useful to accumulate reassuring evidence showing
that sporting successes can follow a night of truly abysmal
sleep. So many factors influence sporting success and some
have just a small impact. Despite the importance of sleep,
gold medals have been won after a night spent tossing and
turning.

Taking my son to play in football matches, it is possible to
see that children who have not long since learned to run are
being scouted by professional sporting clubs. In the UK, it's
not uncommon for five-year-olds to be invited to train with
multiple soccer clubs.* They often still need help going to the
toilet and may not yet be fully competent in using a knife and
fork, but these same children are trained by professionals to
play high-level soccer. The opportunity to learn skills and
tricks and take selfies with football legends may be difficult to
turn down. However, does evening training mean that kids
miss out on the sleep that they need? I think so and, more
generally, the International Olympic Committee published a
consensus statement on youth athletic development noting
among other things that training and competitions can

---

* There are rules about the minimum age that children can be signed
to professional football clubs, but younger children are invited to
train in development programmes.

contribute to sleep deprivation.[40] Missing out on sleep can have negative consequences for multiple areas of functioning and also increase the likelihood of injuries.

I talk to Briony, the mother of seven-year-old Arthur, an outstandingly talented football player, about the challenges of helping her son develop in the sport while respecting his need for sleep. When Arthur plays, it's not unheard of for scouts from multiple Premier League teams to come and watch. They don't want to miss out on signing him if he continues to stand out from the crowd. His coach and parents are often approached after the matches by those interested in recruiting him to train with their team.

Briony explains: 'Our son Arthur loves football and has been attending football training sessions since he was three. Last year Arthur turned seven and was invited to attend three football academies and play for a regular team. He trains up to five times a week and sessions sometimes end as late as 7 p.m. He usually gets home, has something to eat, takes a shower and needs some time to wind down. We find that Arthur sometimes goes to bed after 9.30 p.m. yet still wakes at 6 a.m.' Briony goes on to discuss her dilemma about his football training: 'We worry that Arthur is not getting enough sleep but have decided to continue with the training as he enjoys football so much and is making good progress at school. This year is a decisive year for Arthur in terms of getting signed for a professional team. We feel under a lot of pressure to make the right decisions in order to provide what is best for him in terms of his health and overall wellbeing.'*

Things seem to be going well for Arthur and he is fortunate to have parents who are keen for him to thrive in multiple areas of life, but not all children are so fortunate. Some coaches and parents do not stop to think about the sleep requirements of children, but they should. Adapting training schedules might be one way in which children are given the opportunity to get sufficient sleep.[40] Training during times

---

* I request that should there be competition to sign Arthur, he selects Arsenal, my favourite team.

when children should be preparing for sleep is surely unlikely to be the best way to produce the world's greatest athletes. Those involved in children's football might want to think a little more about the sleep of their young stars if the English are ever going to relive 1966.*

Driving all night: sleep and car accidents

Young adulthood is a time when many learn to drive, creating new-found freedoms. But this freedom is sometimes accompanied by concerning stories about accidents. Young age and inexperience equals a risk for car accidents,[41] but poor sleep and sleepiness are particularly key too. Indeed, there is research to suggest that being young is a particular risk factor for experiencing a sleepiness–related car crash.[42] One explanation for this might be that risky decisions are more common in youth, particularly during adolescence,[43] and also in those who are chronically sleep deprived.[44]

There is no doubt that tiredness kills – drive along the motorway and you will see signs stating just that. It's also clear that people are most vulnerable to car accidents in the early hours of the morning[45] when our body clocks are screaming at us to be asleep. The scientific literature is clear that when we are sleepy we are less vigilant and pay less attention – and crucially our reaction time is slower.[46] The impairment associated with drowsy driving is great and has even been likened to that following the consumption of alcohol or drugs.[47] Worst of all, when we are tired we are more likely to fall asleep at the wheel, which can have catastrophic consequences.

How do we know that sleep causes so many deaths on the roads? We start by excluding other reasons (such as having high levels of alcohol in the body, speeding, poor visibility and phone use). The biggest clues then come from examining

---

* In 1966 England both hosted and won the football World Cup. We are still proud!

tyre marks on the road following an accident. Where there is
no attempt to brake or swerve, it may well be that the driver
was asleep, or otherwise unconscious, before the crash.[48]
'Falling asleep at the wheel is likely to lead to catastrophe,'
says Professor Richard Rowe, a driving behaviour researcher
at the University of Sheffield. 'Even if you don't fall asleep,
your reactions to road hazards will be impaired by sleepiness,
increasing your risk of crashing. This is especially problematic
if you are in the first few years of your driving career.'

The magnitude of the problem is vast and a recent report
estimated that more than 20 per cent of fatal crashes involved
a driver who was drowsy – which amounts to around 6,400
crashes each year in the USA alone.[49] Scientific papers
containing these important messages are typically read by
other scientists and often do not permeate society to the
extent that they should. Instead, sometimes it is the stories of
our lives which make people take note. A 15-year-old me
watched a horrific road crash scene on the news. I was with a
friend who noted that the car in the crash resembled one
owned by another close friend of hers – it was a passing
comment and we thought nothing more of it at the time.
However, the car on the news did belong to her friend.
Coming back home late at night, this lifelong friend alongside
a group of other adolescents all died in the crash. I don't want
to miss the opportunity to remind us all of the power of sleep.
Respect that – and never drive tired.

We can underestimate our own impairment, so know the
signs.[47] Some are obvious – and you should certainly not be
driving if you find yourself yawning, struggling to keep your
eyes open or your head is falling forwards. However, some
signs are less apparent, such as straying out of your lane or
struggling to keep a consistent speed, missing turnings or
signposts or forgetting having driven the past few miles.
When these or other signs of drowsiness occur, you need to
stop and sleep until you no longer feel sleepy. Caffeine can be
useful, but cannot replace sleep itself. Get home safely.

CHAPTER SEVEN

Sleep During the Rush-Hour Years of Our Lives

Adults (26–64 years) recommended 7–9 hours of sleep per 24 hours[1]

The length, timing and organisation of sleep all change dramatically from the time we are born to the time we are approaching middle age. Many would assume that by adulthood everything would be quite settled, and perhaps in some ways it is. Our sleep stages are established and lots of the problems we may have experienced in the past are gone. For the most part, we are no longer arguing with our parents about bedtime, wetting the bed or struggling to fall asleep at an appropriate hour. But then adulthood isn't always an oasis of beige. This stage of life can bring new experiences and challenges. There may be relationship make-ups and break-ups, pregnancies, parenthood and new work responsibilities. Just as the way we sleep might influence all of these things, it also works vice versa. Sleep patterns and problems can differ dramatically between us too, with the sleep of one person varying greatly from that of another.

As we move away from early adulthood, certain features of our sleep remain consistent. For example, it is still recommended that we sleep for seven to nine hours per night. But, of course, there are differences between adults too. Michelle Obama may not sleep in the same way as Barack Obama and these differences are likely to be related to multiple factors. For example, there have been reports that women tend to sleep longer than men.[2] It's not all good news for Mrs Obama though as, despite this longer sleep, women are also more likely than men to report insomnia – a difference that appears to get stronger with age.[3,*]

Sleep may differ between those residing in different countries too and whereas I fall asleep on a mattress on a bedframe, some of those living in Japan will sleep on a tatami mat on the floor. There are other variations too – the inhabitants of some countries, including Spain, Italy, Greece and Mexico may take a siesta. People living in the UK, France and the USA typically do not. This can result in a very different working day and Emilio, the father from Spain whom we met in Chapter 3, describes his work day as starting at 9 a.m. and running until 2 p.m. when he goes home for lunch. He tells me: 'Lunch is the main meal of the day, which for some people can influence having a siesta. A heavy meal plus heat in the summer can all lead to needing a rest.' Emilio returns to work from 4 p.m. to 8 p.m., only getting home to eat dinner at around 9 p.m. or 10 p.m. He ends by saying: 'Here in Spain, the singing competition *The Voice* starts on TV at 10 p.m. and finishes after midnight.' By contrast, my own work day usually starts around 8 a.m. and continues in a single chunk, with the odd drink or snack at my desk, until I stop at around 6 p.m. to make my kids their dinner and start their bedtime routine. If I were to watch *The Voice* UK, I know I could be in bed by 10 p.m.

Sleep length might differ too. A study collecting data through an app suggested that the Dutch get the most sleep, while those from Singapore get the least[2] and we Brits get slightly more than most. But different studies provide different conclusions. For example, a further study led by an insurance company reported that Brits are actually most likely to report not getting enough sleep.[4] While 37 per cent of Brits considered this to be the case, people from India were least likely to make this claim, with only 9 per cent saying they get insufficient sleep. Before interpreting such results it is important to note that participants included in studies of this type might not be representative of the countries in which

---

* While group differences have been reported, there are also large individual differences among women and among men.

they live. Those with poor sleep may be more likely to download a sleep app in the first place, for example. If samples are not representative, it can be difficult to know what to conclude from studies of this type.

So, although precise international differences in sleep patterns are not entirely clear, if differences do exist, why might that be? Certainly, there could be cultural differences including the number of hours we are expected to work and the different pressures we might experience. Differences between countries regarding daylight hours and seasons may also play a role, and sunrise and sunset have been found to influence wake-up time, for example.[2,5] This is noteworthy as the daylight experienced by people living in different countries can differ dramatically – those in Lapland, Finland, will receive very few hours of daylight during the winter but almost continuous daylight during the summer. By contrast, those in Bogota, Colombia, experience around 12 hours of daylight all year around.

Within countries socioeconomic factors play a role and those who are socioeconomically disadvantaged are more vulnerable to getting less sleep or that of poorer quality.[6] To find out more, I meet with Dr Michael Grandner (mentioned in Chapter 1). He explains: 'Sleep exists at this interesting nexus – on one side you have all of the important physiologic processes that sleep plays important roles in. Like metabolism, immune function and emotion regulation. And on the other side you have all of those elements of the social and physical environment that impact our lives. Things like work, home, neighbourhood and family. Sleep plays a critical role for health yet is shaped by these important factors. If we are going to take sleep seriously as an aspect of health, we need to help people gain some control over their sleep in the context of busy, stressed-out lives that can often feel very out of control.'

Insomnia and the city

Although we have waved goodbye to many of the childhood sleep problems by the time we reach adulthood, some of these remain and others appear for the very first time. One lurking issue is insomnia – a common and torturous complaint. Any book on sleep that did not discuss this ailment would be failing its brief. We've probably all had sleepless nights, whether involving anxiety before a big event, sorrow because of a loss, or just too many thoughts racing around our heads as a consequence of a busy life. But occasional instances aside, what happens when sleepless nights turn into a recurrent problem that continues for months at a time and begins to affect our lives intolerably? Insomnia may have taken hold.

Try sharing this all-consuming experience with soundly sleeping friends – and occasionally even doctors – and they sometimes lack understanding. But, this muted response by others reflects the lack of public awareness about this disorder rather than an overreaction of the sufferer. This problem was recently brought to public awareness by the *Sex and the City* actress Kim Cattrall, who pulled out of a play she was due to perform in at a London theatre.[7] The media were confused and assumed that she must have cancer. What was going on? Why had such a hard-working, reliable actress withdrawn from a starring role at such short notice? In fact, she had been suffering from debilitating insomnia – which she described as 'a three-ton gorilla on ... [her] chest' and which had become 'a tsunami' in her life. After taking some time off to get better, she shared her experience. Her brave stance made a difference, and soon after she had publicly discussed her situation, I received an email from someone who was experiencing a similar sleep problem and was now looking for help. So why did Cattrall, and why do so many millions of others like her worldwide, suffer from insomnia and why does it not just go away?

Why does insomnia come and stay?

In Cattrall's case, her insomnia might have been initiated by the 'perfect storm' of struggling with the grief caused by losing her father, anxiety about a new show and experiencing hormonal changes due to her stage of life. Both personal experience and theories of insomnia support the idea that big and stressful events in our lives can trigger insomnia.

Models of this disorder highlight other factors too. Among the leading theories is the 3P model of insomnia, which focuses on predisposing, precipitating and perpetuating factors. This was proposed in the 1980s by the late Art Spielman, who spent much of his career working at Cornell University. The first P refers to **predisposing** factors. What could predispose us to insomnia? A genetic vulnerability, for example, could be important in this disorder developing. This helps to explain why some people are more likely to become sleepless than others.

The second P refers to **precipitating** factors, which may trigger the onset of insomnia. These could include a big life event such as a job loss, a death of a loved one, financial stresses or final exams. People with predisposing factors may be more vulnerable to developing insomnia in the face of precipitating factors.

The final P focuses on **perpetuating** factors – those that feed the insomnia and keep it alive once it has arrived. These could include becoming overly fixated on sleep and worried about it to the extent that it actually stops us from nodding off. We might behave in a way that reinforces the sleep problem. Constantly checking the clock to see how long we have been awake is one sure way to ruin a good night's sleep. Those with predisposing factors may be more vulnerable to developing patterns that feed the insomnia, such as ruminating on the precipitating factors, for example.

Around the start of the millennium, two widely respected sleep researchers, professors Allison Harvey from the University of California, Berkeley (mentioned in the prologue), and Colin Espie, from the University of Oxford, independently developed new models of insomnia. Both flagged the importance of the way that we think in developing and maintaining this sleep disorder.[8,9] These cognitive models of insomnia were similar in their focus and were published in the same year (2002). Here I focus on Harvey's model. Some features of this model can be used to provide an example of how our thinking may be important in the development and maintenance of insomnia. The model begins by considering the way we may react to a night of poor sleep. Instead of forgetting about it and writing it off, we may start to worry about our inability to sleep well – perhaps dreading the night ahead. This can make us feel wound up – which is not great for nodding off. Instead of sleeping well the next night we may lie in bed monitoring our bodies – 'do I feel tired?', 'are my muscles tense?'. We might also monitor everything around us ('I've been lying here awake for a whole hour – and I know it because I've watched every clock stroke'). This can result in an exaggeration of the problem, and we may think that our sleep is much worse than it actually is, or that we just can't cope with it.

We may then attempt to resolve our sleep problem by changing our behaviour in order to sleep better. For example, we may try harder to control what we are thinking about when lying in bed, refusing to let stressful thoughts enter our head. But this can backfire dramatically and result in us giving greater attention to the thoughts we are so keen to avoid. As an illustration, try this experiment. Set your alarm for one minute and think about anything you like except for a chimp wearing a cowboy hat.

Not so easy. You thought about that chimp, right? So trying to block out thoughts isn't always a good strategy.

Another technique that sometimes backfires is going to bed early to catch up on lost sleep. This may result in lying in bed when we are not yet ready to sleep and staying awake for an even longer period. Our anxiety increases as a result and thanks to these counterproductive behaviours we may be on our way to developing a real problem with our sleep.

One feature of Harvey's cognitive model that deserves attention is the idea that monitoring sleep can cause or maintain problems. This is concerning, given the recent popularity of personal sleep monitors. People in their thousands now track their sleep using commercially available wristbands or phone apps that use accelerometers or sounds to draw conclusions about movement. People with these devices sometimes go to bed eagerly awaiting information about the time they spend sleeping and the quality of their sleep. Moreover, concerns have been flagged about the ability of some of these commercial products to accurately estimate the amount that someone sleeps[10-12] or the time they spend in certain stages.[13] This is consistent with some of the feedback I've received from people using these products, such as the young man who claimed that his device showed that he pretty much 'never gets deep sleep' and the middle-aged lady who revealed that she 'sleeps like an 80-year-old'. Refinement of such products is ongoing and it is clear that their potential is great and could come to revolutionise sleep research, providing experts with a cheap way to measure the sleep of a huge number of participants. Until then, it might be best not to take the results as gospel. Those who struggle to sleep in particular might want to think carefully about the potential implications of bringing these products into their lives.

Other characterisations of insomnia include the hyper-arousal model. This includes a stronger emphasis on biological factors, while at the same time acknowledging the importance of psychological ones.[14] Discussing this model, Professor Dieter Riemann from Freiburg University draws upon a large body of literature to demonstrate that many of those who suffer from insomnia appear to experience hyperarousal. In other words, they show signs of feeling wound up and on edge during both the day and night. It's not that big, stressful events in our lives are not important in leading to insomnia. Instead, these events can leave us wound up even after the stressful events in our lives have passed and it's this hyperarousal that causes problems sleeping. We might feel tired, but we also feel wired. This is especially true for those who are at the greatest genetic risk.

What's more, instead of seeing our bedroom as an oasis of calm – an ideal backdrop for drifting off – we might have got into the pattern of associating our bedroom, or indeed bedtime, with feeling stressed and alert. This means that the hyperarousal and subsequent sleep problems can continue even after the stressful events in our lives have passed. When I ask Riemann to elaborate on this model, he tells me:

'Actually, the idea of hyperarousal as a pathophysiological relevant factor for insomnia goes back centuries. It was Michael Perlis in 1997 with his neurocognitive model of insomnia who highlighted that increased frequencies in the fast range of sleep EEG might signal hyperarousal.' Riemann goes on to talk about how this theory has developed over time: 'Work over the last 20 years has brought the psychological data about hyperarousal into contact with neurobiological data. Neuroimaging data, for example, shows that hyperarousal is not just a subjective experience of being unable to shut down, but it is also reflected in increased brain activity during the 24-hour day in people with chronic insomnia.'

Another conceptualisation of insomnia is the metacognitive model proposed by Jason Ong, an associate professor of neurology based at Northwestern University Feinberg School of Medicine in Chicago.[15] Metacognition is sometimes described as 'thinking about thinking'. This could involve awareness that some of our thoughts about sleep are making the problem worse. Trying not to think about that chimp is making us overly occupied by it! This model builds on cognitive models before it, suggesting that the way we interact with our thoughts about sleep may be important. Practical suggestions from this model include that we should not try to change the way we are thinking. Instead, it can be helpful to change our relationship with these thoughts. It can be useful for someone to become aware of the thoughts they are having about their sleep and how these may perpetuate the problems that they are experiencing. Instead of trying to block these out, it can be valuable merely to observe them, and to let the thoughts move in and out of our heads like a breeze through the branches of a tree. Instead of interacting with our thoughts, or wishing them away, we could simply be aware of them, letting them enter and exit our lives without judgement. Such mindfulness-based interventions have been shown to be helpful for multiple aspects of our well-being including our sleep.[16,17] Ong explains to me: 'Rather than forcing sleep or getting absorbed in trying to fix the sleep problem, some people might benefit from letting go and just being present with whatever is happening. This approach to sleep-related thoughts is called mindfulness and research has shown that it can be effective in improving sleep quality.'

Each of these models contributes to our overall understanding of insomnia: the genes that we are born with increase our vulnerability to developing insomnia; stressful life events can trigger episodes; high arousal levels are incompatible with sound sleep, and our behaviours and thinking (including metacognition) can perpetuate problems.

How to make it go away: our thoughts and behaviours

In the case of Cattrall, her insomnia resolved thanks to receiving cognitive behavioural therapy for insomnia (or CBT-I). Guidelines produced by the American College of Physicians have declared this to be the very best first line of treatment for chronic cases of insomnia in adults.[18] Conclusions were based on evidence from the most rigorous and unbiased studies – referred to as 'randomised controlled trials' – and the guidelines are relevant to all clinicians regardless of where they are practising. So, what does this CBT-I treatment involve?

Perhaps unsurprisingly, given the name of the intervention, cognitions (or thoughts) that may be causing or maintaining sleep problems are challenged and corrected. For example, the person with insomnia may be educated about the science of sleep – with the aim of reversing dysfunctional beliefs. Perhaps someone feels that they always need eight hours of slumber to function well, when in fact they may be better suited to seven (experiencing less disturbed sleep and functioning optimally during the day)? Telling them so could avoid unnecessary hours lying wide awake in bed. They may also be taught techniques that have the potential to aid restful sleep, such as savouring, a process that involves taking time to consider a special memory from the past or an event in the future.[19,20] So, instead of lying in bed ruminating about a bad day at work, they might want to relive a special time in their life or think ahead to that trip to the Bahamas they have planned.

There is also, as the name would suggest, a behavioural component to CBT-I. Relaxation techniques can be used to help the patient unwind before bed. Sleep hygiene can also be useful. This might include avoiding coffee or contact with electronic devices after a certain time, as well as making the sleeping environment as dark as possible. Behaviours that are causing or maintaining insomnia can also be corrected using 'stimulus control therapy'. Here people receiving treatment might try to control the associations they have with a stimulus. In the case of insomnia, the stimulus might be 'bedtime and the bedroom' and the association might be 'stress'. With stimulus control therapy the aim is to undo these associations so that bedtime and the bedroom are associated with peace and sleep instead. If they are not tired, they are told not to go to bed. If they wake up in the night and are unable to sleep, they are told to get out of bed and go into another room. They should only go to bed when tired and only spend time in bed when they are ready to sleep. Following this technique, over time they begin to associate the bedroom with relaxation and sleep rather than sleepless nights.

Another technique used within CBT-I, and one that is often considered beneficial in addressing insomnia, is sleep restriction therapy. This involves restricting the amount of time in bed in order to avoid spending time in bed awake. So, if they spend eight hours in bed, but just seven hours sleeping, they may be advised to reduce time in bed to seven hours. People with insomnia are effectively concentrating their sleep so that it is more efficient and they are more likely to get the type of sleep that they need. This technique works because when sleep is restricted, the drive for it increases. That means that people are more likely to spend the limited time they now have in bed fast asleep – rather than awake tossing and turning. This has the additional benefit of weakening the link between bed and wakefulness, and strengthening that between the bed and sleep. This technique is not always easy though, as when exhausted, it can be some challenge to limit the hours spent in bed.

Take, for example, the case of Roger, a government employee who suffers from severe and long-term insomnia. He recently undertook an online course of CBT-I. He reported that after a week of terrible sleep, where he was getting about four hours a night, he started sleeping for longer periods. This coincided with being offered advice that he should restrict his sleep. He could not quite find it in himself to limit the sleep he had been craving for so long so ignored this advice and abandoned the course. Weeks later his insomnia returned and he felt frustrated with himself for having chosen a single dose of sleep over the advice that he had been offered to help deal with the problems over the long term.

For those who think that CBT-I might be for them, the next step is to find an expert who can deliver this treatment. There are not as many experts in this technique as there should be, so this is not always easy. For this reason, there has been great excitement about recently developed online methods of delivery, such as that which Roger tried.

According to Espie (see p. 175), from the University of Oxford, who is also co-founder of Big Health, a digital medicine company: 'Making CBT available on the web and mobile phones has the advantage of being "scalable". That is, it could be there to help immediately, for anyone who might benefit from it. The goal is to make "digital medicine" (dCBT) as easy to access as pharmaceutical medicine (sleeping pills).' Others agree about the potential of online treatments and it has even been suggested that these resources should be offered in the workplace, given that they are considered to be cost-effective in reducing lost productivity caused by insomnia.[21]

But others have flagged concerns surrounding the removal of face-to-face contact. It has also been pointed out that these techniques need to be thoroughly tested to show that they work well.[22] Espie agrees with this latter point: 'Of course dCBT has to be proven to work ... we have emphasised the importance of conducting extensive scientific trials on [our online programme] Sleepio. We are not the only people to be doing this of course, but we remain determined that the evidence for dCBT is rigorous as well as transformative in terms of healthcare provision.' Thinking about the bigger picture, he adds: 'Incidentally, I also believe that digital medicine will in time become integrated with expert in-person clinical services; meaning that clinicians can focus their time and resources on the situations that most need their personal attention, while at the same time using digital tools to support their work and enable them to work more efficiently and effectively.'

CBT-I is the best treatment we have for insomnia, but it does not work for everyone. In the case of Roger, a few months after his aborted CBT attempt, he declared that he'd finally been fixed by self-medicating with 'CBD'. Had he got his acronyms muddled? Apparently not. CBD (cannabidiol) is one of the two main active components of cannabis (the other being THC (tetrahydrocannabinol), which is the part that gets you high). Roger purchased the oil (legally) from his local health food shop and merrily dropped some CBD oil into cashew milk each night before bed. He reported falling into a deep slumber and waking up feeling refreshed. Despite Roger's enthusiasm for CBD, self-medicating holds risks and is not recommended. Furthermore, there have not been many good-quality studies examining the effects – and those studies that have investigated the effects of cannabis more generally and its active components on sleep have produced mixed results.[23] In Roger's case the CBD eventually stopped working and he was prescribed a very low dose of an antidepressant to help him relax. They currently appear to be working well. But why was he not prescribed sleeping pills? Do they work? Are they safe?

Medication for insomnia

Compared with CBT-I, there is much weaker evidence to support the use of sleeping pills for treating insomnia. Sleeping pills include both benzodiazepines and 'Z-drugs' and should only be prescribed for a very short time, after a good deal of consideration and in instances where CBT-I has failed to bring about improvements.[18] These drugs have a calming effect by boosting the impact of the inhibitory neurotransmitter GABA (mentioned in Chapter 1) in the brain. These drugs can help us nod off – so may sound tempting to someone suffering from a serious bout of insomnia. However, they don't produce sleep as we know it. Instead, they bring about a poor substitute. Benzodiazepines, for example, result in less deep sleep and REM sleep, leaving us in a light state of sleep.[24] No wonder we can wake up after taking these pills feeling lousy. What's more, they do nothing to treat the underlying cause of insomnia – so provide a sticky plaster, which at best holds things together in the short term. If these drugs are taken for over a few weeks tolerance can develop, meaning we need more and more of them to do the job. Dependence can also result, with unpleasant withdrawal symptoms when these drugs are eventually stopped.

A combination of desperation over lack of sleep and the availability of certain drugs has sometimes resulted in catastrophic consequences. This might have been the case with the tragic death of the musician Michael Jackson. He had traces of benzodiazepines in his body and also had the drug propofol in his system, which appeared to have caused him to stop breathing.[25]

Sleep researchers and the wider world were shocked. In particular, there was concern that he had been given propofol, which is not a sleep aid but a general anaesthetic. If you remember back to Chapter 1, it was pointed out that sleep is somewhat different from anaesthesia. If we were to try operating on someone who was asleep, the difference would become clear pretty quickly. As Charles Czeisler, professor of sleep medicine at Harvard Medical School, pointed out during a trial, propofol disrupts the sleep cycle and does not provide REM sleep, meaning that while someone given this drug may wake up feeling rested, they may actually be becoming increasingly sleep deprived.[26] In the case of

Michael Jackson, this could help to explain symptoms before his death, which were reported in the media to include becoming paranoid, losing weight and no longer being able to remember the words and dances to his era-defining music. If he was given these drugs because he was desperate for sleep, it is incredibly sad that he was not able to get the appropriate help.

Sleeping with someone

When studied in a sleep laboratory, the chances are we are assessed alone. There is no consideration of what our partners do during the night, which doesn't make a lot of sense, as over half of adults sleep with a partner.[27] The fact that our partners may go to bed an hour or so later than us, wake an hour before us, snore and hog the duvet is totally ignored. However, don't these things have a huge impact on our own sleep?

Perhaps we need to spend a little more time thinking about sleep as a communal activity. After all, it's been argued that one benefit of our circadian rhythm is to keep us awake during the day and asleep at night. This way, communities are encouraged – with people doing the same thing at the same time.[28,*] Just as universal similarities in circadian rhythms may have led to the formation of social groups, it is easy to imagine that differences between people in this timing (an owl sleeping with a lark) could lead to relationship problems.

Rakesh, a middle-aged city worker, discusses with me some problems that he and his wife have with their sleep. 'It's funny,' he tells me. 'Neither of us has a problem separately,

---

* It has been noted elsewhere in this book that differences in sleep timing can also help to support communities (with people awake to look over the group at different times). However, these differences are relatively subtle and are still within a general diurnal pattern of being primarily awake during the day and asleep at night.

but we have a big problem together.' He goes on to describe that his wife goes to bed earlier than he does and wakes up later. She is naturally a long sleeper, whereas he gets by on just a little sleep. 'The problem is due to our asynchronous sleep patterns. I tiptoe to bed hours after she has turned in, but always manage to wake her up. She wakes up and starts worrying about really random things and asks me for advice while I am half asleep. I talk nonsense and both of us get annoyed.'

How a partner's sleep can drive you to despair

Other aspects of sleep can also result in problems between couples. Snoring and sleep apnoea can impair sleep and life quality for more than just the sufferer.[29,30] Sleep researchers have pointed out that snoring can be louder than a road drill.[31] Yes, really! Other sleep disorders can cause relationship problems too – sleeping next to someone whose legs won't stop running does not make for a restful night of sleep either. At the more extreme end, being punched at night by a sleeping partner with REM sleep behaviour disorder will really test one's tolerance. Even the smallest thing our partner does can disturb our sleep. Whether you prefer a hard or soft mattress, a duvet or bed sheets, or like to snuggle up or sleep in a star shape, sleeping as a pair may involve negotiation.

Call the lawyers: seeking a sleep divorce

So, it seems that sleep problems can contribute to relationship problems – but what can be done about it? That depends on what exactly is going on. If partners' sleep timing is incompatible, perhaps larks and owls could attempt to slightly shift their sleep timings so they become more aligned. It's also useful to seek help for sleep disorders when they occur. Sleep apnoea, for example, can be reduced by a technique called 'continuous positive airway pressure', or CPAP. This involves wearing a mask through which air is blown to help maintain the appropriate pressure in the airways. Some report that this makes them look and feel like Darth Vader. For those who are not convinced that this treatment is for them, less well-established treatments have been proposed too. There's even some evidence to suggest that didgeridoo training during the day might provide certain benefits for those with moderate sleep apnoea – perhaps by strengthening the muscles of the upper airways![32] But continuous positive airway pressure remains the treatment of choice and can improve life, not only for a patient but for their bed partner too.[29,30]

Even education has the potential to help. Just knowing that there is a biological basis for our partner staying up until 2 a.m. before an early start can help avoid conflict. Recently, my friend Tina told me that she and her husband had bickered for some time over their very different sleep schedules. She would stay up until at least 2 a.m., while he would have been asleep for some time by then. He'd then get up many hours before she did. One day when driving, Tina's husband stumbled upon a radio broadcast on circadian rhythms by the eminent scientists professors Russell Foster, Debora Skene and Steven Jones. They were discussing the biological basis of the circadian system.[28] Overnight her husband's frustrated eye rolls morphed into sympathetic glances, and for the first time in their multi-decade relationship he began to accept her quirky sleep pattern.

Of course, there is also the most extreme solution – divorce. Before calling in the lawyers, perhaps a sleep divorce is a better way forward. More and more people are choosing to leave the marital bed and sleep alone. If it means a better night's sleep for both and an improved relationship, why not embrace it? This is undoubtedly not for everyone, and some people respond to the suggestion of a sleep divorce with the same hurt as if the real thing has been proposed. When I suggest a separate sleeping arrangement to Rakesh the aforementioned city worker, he smiles. 'Funnily enough, my wife always ends up sleeping in the spare room. She gets sick of lying awake while I'm asleep and goes to lie somewhere else. Having said that, neither of us like the idea of starting the night in separate beds. Not sure why, but it just doesn't feel right.' Talking this through with Dr Wendy Troxel, a sleep researcher who specialises in couples' sleep, she notes: 'It's important for couples to realise that there is not a one-size-fits-all approach to sleeping arrangements. Couples need to determine what works best for them and have a healthy dialogue about it with their partner.'

For those people who think the ultimate solution to avoiding a bad night's sleep is to sod the sleep divorce and go for an actual divorce, think again. It seems that those who are divorced sleep worse than others.[27] In considering why this may be the case, the stress and conflict associated with divorce could play a role. But there could also be lots of other reasons, and perhaps tricky life circumstances could increase our chances of both getting divorced and sleeping poorly too. Recent data suggests that marital therapy results in better sleep – although unfortunately, ladies, this was only found to be the case for husbands.[33]

Sleep and pregnancy

Many people have children at some point in their lives and this typically occurs during adulthood. Even before conception, it is possible that sleep plays a role, and studies have linked sleep length or quality to the size of a man's testicles, sperm count and quality.[34,35] It has also been proposed that female fertility could be associated with sleep, with one possible mechanism being that insomnia causes the body stress that impacts upon fertility via an effect on reproductive hormones.[36] The authors of a review on this topic hypothesise that disrupted sleep could reflect something threatening in our lives. This might make an associated reduction in fertility an evolutionarily adaptive response by avoiding bringing a baby into a dangerous environment. Further research is needed to confirm links and test hypotheses – and, if sleep quality and fertility are linked in important ways, to see whether improving sleep could be a method by which fertility can be enhanced.

When pregnancy does occur, just by looking at women who are about to give birth, it's clear that sleep might be tricky. For those in doubt, perhaps stick a football up your pyjama top when you go to bed and see what that does for your sleep and fatigue levels the next day. In addition to the discomfort caused by the bulk of having a living thing and its kit inside your belly, the pregnancy hormones oestrogen and progesterone, and the stress that so often occurs with this period of life, can also mess with your sleep. This is all borne out in the literature.[37] Women may struggle with the quality of their sleep from as early as their first trimester, when they also begin to sleep for longer periods than previously.[38] It can also be difficult getting comfortable and multiple night wakings can occur, sometimes because of the need to urinate.[37] Wide-ranging sleep problems may arise during pregnancy, and include insomnia, restless legs syndrome and sleep-disordered breathing. Some report the saving grace of daytime naps.

Improving maternal comfort during pregnancy is important. But, just as essential, it seems that poor maternal sleep during pregnancy could be associated with undesirable outcomes such as the birth of a premature baby or postnatal depression – although authors caution that further studies are necessary before clear conclusions can be reached.[39,40] The mechanisms by which this might occur appear to be via the body's stress response, and changes in the immune response and inflammation in the body.[41] Overall, it would seem that disrupted sleep during pregnancy deserves clinical attention.

Sleep and parenthood

Pregnancy can spell troubled sleep, but the woes are unlikely to cease when the bundle of joy arrives with a three-hour around-the-clock waking schedule. Then the sleep deprivation really kicks off. No first-time parent is really prepared for what is about to descend. A mother might have longed for the end of pregnancy, imagining a time when she will be in a physical state to get more sleep. In reality there is often no time to recover from the challenges of pregnancy and birth. Instead, parents are often starting a marathon of further disturbed nights.

Research backs up just how sleep deprived and exhausted parents are in the first months that follow the birth, with new parents experiencing more disturbed sleep, sleepiness and sleepiness-related difficulties compared with childless couples.[42] A report from a small study found that when babies are first born, fathers got less sleep than mothers.[43] But, that is not to imply that mothers had it easy: they slept for less time during the night – and had to compensate by sleeping during the day.* Sleep deprivation and disruption make new parenthood a vulnerable time – potentially putting them at risk of driving accidents[44] and other problems that can ensue as a result of insufficient sleep.

As the years roll on, it might be that introducing a child to the world could produce the greatest changes to a mother's sleep length. In a study of more than 5,800 adults, presented at a conference in Boston and reported in the *Chicago Tribune*, having children was associated with insufficient sleep in women, but not in men.[45] Before assuming that this reflects lazy fathers not pulling their weight, sleep expert Mindell (mentioned in Chapter 2) commented that we should consider other explanations. For example, it is possible that men are more likely to experience short sleep even before having children, so having children doesn't result in such a big change in their sleep. This sits well with data from almost 180,000 workers.[46] Overall, males were slightly more likely to report sleeping less than seven hours a night (38 per cent) than females (35 per cent).

---

* An additional study also found that during the early stages of a baby's life mothers got more sleep than fathers.[42] However, again, it was not a case of mothers getting the better end of the bargain – they were found to have more disrupted sleep, with more night-time waking.

These general trends do not capture individual family circumstances, and when we look at single-parent families (and particularly when that single parent is a woman) they are especially likely to miss out on their slumber.[47] Overall, it seems that whether we are a mother or a father, we are unlikely to be winning the sleep lottery any time soon. When we lock horns with a partner over sleep, it may be useful to keep in mind that they are possibly struggling as much as we are. This is easier said than done, when sleep deprived and on a short fuse.

The problem with the sleep of new parents is often twofold. Not only are parents sleep deprived, but when they do catch some Zs they may experience dire sleep, being woken repeatedly during the night. The late Professor Sadeh (mentioned in Chapter 5) and his colleagues wanted to investigate the effects of this disturbed sleep on mood and attention.[48] The idea here was that being woken during the night in an experiment might mimic what goes on in families, where parents are repeatedly disturbed at night in order to do something – such as feed an infant or change a nappy – before being permitted to sleep once more. Actually, multiple night awakenings are common outside the parenting context and medical professionals on call and pet owners may all be woken repeatedly at night. The participants in this study were allocated either to a sleep restriction group, where they were asked to sleep for no longer than four hours during the night; or to a night waking group, in which they were allowed to spend eight hours in bed, but were interrupted four times – every hour and a half – and asked to complete a 10-minute task before returning to sleep. Interestingly, the researchers found that interrupted sleep appeared to be as problematic as getting hardly any sleep. Participants who had short sleep or broken sleep showed poorer attention and greater depression and fatigue compared with when they were assessed after sleeping normally. The fact that there were no differences between those who had experienced very little sleep and those who had experienced longer sleep but were repeatedly woken, helps to explain why new parents suffer so greatly with their sleep, even if they manage to catch up on their Zs during the day.

Parents' sleep: When does it return to its former glory?

In addition to the surprise of just how vile sleep deprivation is, parents are often shocked by its duration. Pregnancy is tough, the first few months with a newborn can be challenging and a large proportion of children are still waking in the night at three years of age. But what lies beyond? There is not a great deal of research examining this, but what there is tends to emphasise the reciprocal nature of sleep within the family – children's sleep patterns affect parents and vice versa.[49] Overall, in one study, it was estimated that employed parents miss out on a total of 645 hours of sleep while raising a child for 18 years compared with those who do not have children.[50] For someone who needs 8 hours of sleep each night, that's equivalent to more than 80 entire nights of sleep lost – and as a parent, I can tell you it feels a whole lot more. The good news, however, is that it seems parents get slightly more sleep as the years roll by and babies turn into toddlers, then children, teenagers and finally adults. In fact, parents of adult children did not report shorter sleep than those without children.

Anecdotally, however, a parent's sleep never returns to its former glory. Those with children find that there's always something getting in the way of sleep: a wet bed, an ill child, a frantic trip to A&E, a small person found unexpectedly nestling against you. Even parents of adolescents and young adults report lying awake anxiously awaiting the safe return of their precious offspring. Perhaps elderly parents still worry about their middle-aged children at night?

So, why might parents sleep more poorly than before their children were born, even once the children are a bit older? One possibility is that being on red alert may be the crux of the problem. Being aroused or attentive is at complete odds with being asleep (we can't be vigilant and asleep at the same time). However, as a parent, there is always a part of me that remains alert to my children's needs. A cough from down the hallway can be enough to wake me these days. It can feel as if part of my brain is awake, guarding my treasure. Or perhaps I need to stop blaming the children and appreciate that this is partly an age-related issue. It's true that as adults age, our sleep quality sometimes gets worse. So perhaps even without children, there would be another reason to lie awake at night worrying.

Parents SOS (save our sleep)

Given what we know about sleep and mental health, it should perhaps come as no surprise that parents of children who don't sleep very well are more likely than those of good sleepers to report stress and depression.[51] If you consider links between disturbed or short sleep and weight gain, neuropsychological functioning and general health, it's also no wonder that the early years of parenting can be among the most challenging of our lives.

The message that sleep deprivation in parents is associated with certain difficulties is perhaps only useful if coupled with a clear message that it is OK for parents to get help. We should capitalise on any resource we may have and consider all options. Help from a kindly grandparent, an expensive nanny, a trip to the doctor or a period off work might all help to carry us through this exhausting time of life.

Sleep and work

For many of us, work is a central component of our adult lives and it is often during this stage of life that careers really begin to kick off in earnest. The amount of time that we might dedicate to work, our work-related stresses, or even the timing of our jobs, can create havoc for our sleep. Headlines reflect this and it's been reported that 'Night work "throws body into chaos"',[52] for example. But headlines also underscore the idea that losing sleep is no good thing for our work performance either, with claims that 'Sleep loss "starts arguments at work"'[53] and of 'Sleep deprivation damaging business'.[54]

Evidence of this sleep–work incompatibility is all around us. Liam, a local friend in his 50s, invited me in for a cup of tea. We partook in the usual neighbourhood chit-chat before turning our conversation to work. I mentioned I was writing this book and Liam recounted his own experiences about sleep. He had really struggled with sleep deprivation when his youngest son was born. He was so exhausted that he would arrive at work having forgotten how he'd got there. He simply had no memory of his drive (which, you might remember from the section on sleep and driving is a sure sign that you should not be on the road). Having been a highly productive member of staff, he was now plodding through the day barely able to stay awake, feeling like he was existing in some strange fog.

Some jobs

Our sleep can create problems for our working lives but some jobs seem to pose particular risks for our sleep. Talk to someone with a typical London city job in banking or finance, for example, and don't be surprised to find that they work around the clock. After all, 'money never sleeps'. This chimes well with my discussion about sleep with Rakesh, the city worker who discussed his wife's sleep patterns with me earlier in this chapter. Rakesh leaves the house before 6 a.m. every morning and returns after 8 p.m. Describing his journey to work, he tells me: 'I get the 6 a.m. train into Waterloo, after having got changed in the dark so as not to wake the family. I've been known to discover on the train that I'm wearing different coloured trousers to my suit jacket! I'm chronically tired and can't keep my eyes open on my way to work. Lots of people on the train are like that and you see a few people every morning with their head nodding as if they can't stay awake. Some people are completely passed out and I often need to tap people on the shoulder at Waterloo to wake them up, so that they don't stay on the train and end up in Bournemouth! The upside of this is that I start the day feeling like I've done a good deed.'

But it's not just the City that's causing problems. In a survey by the Centers for Disease Control and Prevention in the USA, the prevalence of short sleepers (those sleeping less than seven hours a night) was analysed by occupation.[46] Almost 180,000 people had their jobs split into 22 major categories. Those most likely to report short sleep worked in 'production' (43 per cent), 'healthcare support' (40 per cent), 'healthcare practitioners and technical' (40 per cent) and 'food preparation and serving-related' (40 per cent). Those least likely to report short sleep worked in 'education, training and library' and 'farming, fishing and forestry' (both 31 per cent). Self-reported data incorporates certain limitations, such as whether people working in certain occupations are likely to divulge their insufficient sleep. Nonetheless, such information might aid employers in deciding whether they might particularly need to help their staff prioritise their sleep.

Other jobs may also pose risks and military personnel and veterans may be at risk of insomnia. Insomnia can arise in these people because they have experienced stressful situations or because of an irregularity of sleep patterns and difficulties associated with adjusting to life at home following a tour of service.[55] This is problematic, given that sleep problems can exacerbate other difficulties common in this population, such as post-traumatic stress disorder and depression.

Then there are astronauts! How on earth (or rather *off* earth) do astronauts get 40 winks? When in space there is no gravity so surely it's a challenge to get bedded down. Then, if orbiting the Earth, there are unusual patterns of light and dark, caused by the sun rising and setting repeatedly within a 24-hour period. The temperature and noise pollution is not always conducive to optimal sleep either. Surely these things make it impossible to get any slumber? Apparently not. Astronauts climb into a sleeping bag and harness themselves to the floor, wall or ceiling when they hit the sack so that they don't float off and bump into things. They often have their own sleeping stations, or pods, representing bedrooms. This all sounds rather uncomfortable and may help to explain why, in space, astronauts report getting poor sleep, suffering from insomnia and using sleeping pills.[56] Excitement associated with the job is unlikely to result in great sleep either – and after walking on the moon, Buzz Aldrin apparently obtained just a couple of hours of sleep.[57] Neil Armstrong got absolutely none. But could sleeping in space bring certain advantages too? Instead of having to work hard to find the perfect mattress and pillows, and to get into an agreeable position, there is no gravity so bodies are naturally supported. Perhaps aspects of this sleep environment are not so bad and could even provide one up on the other popular sleep locations, including waterbeds and hammocks.

Doctors and nurses are another group whose job requirements may be incompatible with the sleep they are permitted. They literally have our lives in their hands and must be able to tap their vast knowledge quickly, make careful decisions, yet be personable. However, their long working hours must make this challenging at times. In fact, results of one study showed that a night of missed sleep can lead to greater impairment in performance than drinking alcohol to the legal driving limit.[58] In this study, there were two conditions. In one, participants were sleep deprived for 28 hours. In the other they were given drinks containing alcohol at a steady rate until their blood alcohol level hit the 0.10 per cent mark. Throughout both conditions, hand-eye coordination was assessed repeatedly using a computerised task. It was found that performance on the task decreased progressively in both conditions. When the authors tried to quantify this, they found that the reduction in performance after having been sleep deprived for 24 hours was equivalent to having a blood-alcohol concentration of 0.10 per cent, which is quite something, given that the current legal limit for driving in the UK and USA is less than this, at 0.08 per cent. Would one implication of this study be that it might be preferable to be operated on by a surgeon who has enjoyed a glass of wine than one who has missed out on a night's sleep? And even when adequate shut-eye is obtained, the work schedules can be hugely disruptive, with doctors working by night and sleeping by day.[59]

Shift work presents a particular challenge – and not just for medical staff. Light and food, among other things, carefully tune our body clocks to the world around us and the incredible machine that is our body is adjusted perfectly for the day ahead. Now imagine that we give a royal two-fingered salute to common sense and have to stay up all night and sleep during the day instead – perhaps eating a heavy meal in the middle of the night. This is exactly what Guy, a 30-year-old control room worker for a railway company, has to do. He works on a complex six-week rota of early mornings (7 a.m.–3 p.m.), late evenings (3 p.m.–11 p.m.) and nights (7 p.m.–7 a.m.). And he is not alone. Other key workers in our society, like our policemen and pilots, work gruelling schedules too.

At what cost?

So, it seems that our work can affect our sleep and our sleep can affect our work, but what are the costs involved? Getting signed off work with exhaustion is just one way in which sleep can affect our working lives. Costs can also be accrued by poor productivity or rather simply not doing our jobs very well. Thinking back to city workers, a lack of sleep might come with far greater risks than Rakesh's story of workers missing their train stops. Take, for example, the tragic case of Moritz Erhardt, a 21-year-old German who was living in London and completing an internship at a leading bank.[60] By all accounts he was working incredibly long hours, sometimes through the night. He was known to have sent emails at 4 a.m., 5 a.m. and 6 a.m. On 15 August 2013, as he was in the final stages of his internship, he failed to turn up at work. He was later found dead in his shower, having suffered an epileptic fit. Although it is possible that his missed sleep was entirely coincidental to this dreadful event, a lack of sleep and tiredness are known triggers for epileptic seizures. The corporate world's attitude towards sleep needs to change urgently.

Studies have attempted to examine the links between restricted or disrupted sleep and loss of manpower due to accidents and even death. Focusing on insomnia, research led by those at Harvard Medical School asked 4,991 employees with a variety of different jobs about insomnia and other chronic conditions as well as costly workplace accidents or mistakes in the previous year.[61] From the responses, the authors estimated that accidents and errors related to insomnia were more common and associated with greater costs compared with those related to other conditions. They also projected that in the USA there are 274,000 costly workplace accidents that are related to insomnia each year. Although reasons for accidents are often multifaceted, sleep or tiredness have also been mentioned in relation to a number of particularly devastating workplace accidents. These include the Chernobyl nuclear plant disaster where radiation sickness eventually led to multiple deaths; the *Challenger* space shuttle explosion in which seven people died; and the *Exxon Valdez* oil spill where a super-tanker hit a reef, spewing huge quantities of oil and resulting in a wildlife catastrophe.[62]

It seems that missing out on sleep might have significant costs – but how extensive are these? In a recent project by the research institute RAND Europe, it was estimated that insufficient sleep costs $411 billion a year in the USA.[63] That amounts to a whopping 2.28 per cent of GDP! Of course, other countries suffer financially from sleep deprivation too, with the UK estimated to lose around £40 billion each year because of it.

In addition to the financial cost of sleep deprivation and the immediate health risks, it seems that the effects of short sleep over time can be cumulative.[64] This fits well with the finding that working long hours during the middle years of life can have long-lasting effects. One study found that businessmen from Finland who worked long hours and missed out on their Z's were in poorer health more than 20 years later than those who had worked normal hours and got a normal amount of sleep.[65]

Shift work, which is linked with poor sleep quality, appears to have particular ramifications. When I ask Guy, the control room worker on the railway, about life as a shift worker, he tells me: 'Working shifts is like being permanently jetlagged. You don't really appreciate how bad it is until you go back to a 9–5 job. Shift work makes me really quick-tempered, and I only really feel OK again probably five days after finishing my nights and my body clock is getting back to normality.'

So is Guy's experience, and our gut response that shift work comes with risks, supported by the literature? Unfortunately so – shift workers report poorer well-being and mental health than their typically sleeping comrades.[66] They are also more likely than others to experience so many of the things that are dreaded in life: cancer,[67,68] diabetes,[69] heart attacks and strokes.[70] This provides a new meaning to the phrase the 'graveyard shift'.

But why is shift work related to health problems? It is possible that those of us who are vulnerable to health problems are also the ones who end up doing shift work. Perhaps being dealt a tough hand in life has led to limited work choices and increased vulnerability to a range of physical and mental health problems. It's possible that this could explain certain cases. However, this probably wouldn't convince most of us who are unsure that the average doctor or pilot is disadvantaged. Perhaps a more obvious conclusion is that it is the other way around: shift work increases the risk of health problems.

One of the first lessons I was taught as a PhD student, is that it's surprisingly hard to demonstrate that anything is a cause of anything else. There are often multiple alternative explanations that can't be ruled out without a fight. Just because two things are associated, it doesn't mean that one causes the other. After all, it's been shown that between the years of 2000 and 2009, the yearly consumption of mozzarella cheese per capita correlated highly with the yearly number of doctorates awarded in civil engineering – but that is not to suggest that one of these variables is causing the other.* However, in the case of shift work, it may well be that, as with smoking and

---

* For this and other spurious correlations, see the website: www. tylervigen.com/spurious-correlations.

health problems, there is a causal link. The type of evidence that leads us to believe this includes 'dose–response relationships'. Here you find that more of one thing (in this case shift work) is linked to more of another (in this case cancer).[67] Findings such as these leave researchers wide-eyed at their computer screens, acknowledging the importance and implications of what they might be discovering.

More conclusive findings still come from messing with the circadian rhythms of our whiskery friends. Take mice that are vulnerable to developing breast cancer and vary their light–dark cycle week-by-week (in much the same way as that experienced by certain shift workers). You find that they gain weight and develop cancer more quickly than those left on a standard schedule.[71] The research on the links between shift work and cancer has even influenced policy, and in Denmark long-term shift workers who went on to develop breast cancer were compensated by the government.[72] The World Health Organization has also highlighted links between shift work and various health problems and concluded that shift work is a probable carcinogen.

But not all research supports the idea that shift work leads to cancer. Just as scientists were becoming convinced of the causal link between the two, along came a meta-analysis of 10 studies that included a total of 1.4 million women. The researchers examined the link between shift work and breast cancer, finding no association between the two, even in women who had been working shifts for decades.[73] Others have explained the discrepancy between the conclusions of this work and that of others by pointing to methodological differences between reports such as a focus on retired women who may have taken part in shift work many years before; and the possibility that links between shift work and breast cancer are stronger in younger women than older ones.[74] Overall, it would seem that shift work may well be a contributing factor to certain cases of breast cancer or other problems – but why?

If we think back to Captain Obvious and the Clock, it's noteworthy that in addition to the Greenwich-esque clock (situated in the suprachiasmatic nucleus or SCN), different regions of the body are wearing their own time-pieces. Almost every cell in our body has its own clock. When we start to change our patterns, by eating at night, for example, the Greenwich clock may stop calling the shots. In certain cases the mini-clocks in our body, such as those controlling gene expression* in the liver (which gets time cues from our feeding rhythms), can start running out of sync with other areas of the body.[75]

Under normal circumstances, we live in a way that makes the most of our naturally fluctuating levels of alertness, performance, metabolism and sleep drive. But when we sleep by day and work by night, our work schedule, sleep and eating do not fit in with our biology. The darkness hormone melatonin that tells us that it's time to go to sleep is typically released in the evening and is suppressed by light, so sleeping in the day can become tricky. It's noteworthy that melatonin has been implicated in some of the problems that shift workers experience too – such as depression.[66] By sleeping during the day and working at night we're also likely to decrease our exposure to sunshine and thus vitamin D, providing another route by which shift work could leave us weakened.

The effect of shift work on our social lives should not be dismissed either. Remember how, in adolescence, sleep timing might make our youth run out of sync with everyone else in society? Well, the same is true of shift workers, and work of this type could result in decreased opportunities to spend time with the family and enjoy the company of friends, resulting in possible conflict and social isolation.[66] It seems that might be the case to some extent for Guy, the railway control room worker, who tells me: 'For some reason you feel more at home at work than you do at home. Maybe it's because everyone is in the same boat.' The influence of shift work on our social lives might also help to explain why shift workers experience poorer well-being than others.

---

* Or rather controlling the mechanism by which messages in DNA are used to make products such as proteins.

Finally, working shifts could lead to all of these health problems via the negative impact on the quality and length of our kip.[76] This is true of Guy, who tells me: 'While I'm on nights I try my hardest to get at least six to seven hours of sleep in the day, which isn't always possible, and sometimes I get just three to four hours. After my last night shift, I try to get as little sleep as possible, four hours maximum. I also use the powers of alcohol in the evening so I can get to sleep earlier and at a normal time (11 p.m.) – but I'm normally up again through the night anyway.' Talking to Guy more about the train route that he is responsible for, I realise that it overlaps with that on which my own grandad worked. Grandad was a steam-locomotive driver who worked three shifts: the 'early' (6 a.m.–2 p.m.), 'late' (2 p.m.–10 p.m.), and 'night' (10 p.m.–6 a.m.). He dreaded the night shift and had real problems adjusting to the change of sleep pattern, especially during the first couple of days that he was on this shift. He lived opposite the village butcher's shop, where people would meet outside to chew the fat, which would keep him awake. He once expressed his frustration at how this prevented him from sleeping. Everyone knew each other, and the prop of curtains closed should have been more than enough to allow them to realise the consequences of their actions. My grandfather died before his time of a tumour-related illness and I can't help but wonder if things could have been different.

How to reconcile the incompatibility of sleep and work

It appears that sleep and work can pose challenges for one another, but what can be done about this? The nuclear option would be to resign! Before we turn in our resignations in a blaze of financial uncertainty, it might be useful to think back to the differences between us. Take shift work, for example. Some of us seem to crumble after a single late night, whereas others are surprisingly adept at all-night partying. Research supports the idea that some people are better able to cope with shift work than others.[77] A whole host of reasons may be important here, including genetic differences between us. Other factors that seem to help people cope with shift work include being young, male, an evening rather than morning person, low on neuroticism or an extrovert, although not all studies support these conclusions. The type of shift work may also be important, and all shift work was not created equal. Whether it's rotating shifts, permanent night shifts or weekend shifts, for example, can affect the outcome.[78]

So, resignation aside, is there anything else that can be done to reduce the seeming incompatibility between our sleep and our jobs? Is there a way to have it all? In the case of my local friend Liam, who struggled so greatly when his youngest son was born, he started having a recurring and realistic dream that he would have a fatal road accident driving to work. Realising that something was going to give, whether when driving in his car, at work or with his well-being, he was smart enough to know his limitations, so went to the doctor and was signed off work. Away from his job he was able to catch up on the sleep he needed and soon enough returned to work as his highly productive self.

But should it really be entirely down to the individual to find a solution? Surely employers could help too? Some big corporations appear to have woken up to the fact that a rested brain may be a smarter, more creative and productive one. They are doing what they can to respect sleep, with reports of sleeping facilities available at leading companies including Google, PwC and Uber.[79] There are other ways that companies can respect the sleep of their staff too, with certain organisations allowing employees to work from home to avoid long commutes, work flexible hours to let us respect our natural body rhythms and discouraging seemingly endless electronic communication outside of working hours.[80] One company even pays its staff up to $300 a year in bonuses if they sleep![81] Staff can claim $25 for every 20 nights that they report sleeping for seven or more hours.

There have been attempts within the workplace to alter lighting to improve alertness during the day and slumber by night. As discussed in Chapter 4, blue light is able to suppress the darkness hormone melatonin, which tells our bodies that it is time to go to sleep. Blue light has been associated with increased arousal and alertness too – so can be helpful at certain times of the day. Because of this, in one study, lighting was manipulated in the workplace so that workers were given blue-enriched white light for four weeks and standard white light for four weeks.[82] As expected, the blue-enriched white light led to multiple benefits, including increased alertness and concentration, mood and performance. It was also associated with lower levels of daytime sleepiness, evening fatigue and irritability. Added to the bargain, participants reported better sleep quality at night too.

And what advice is there for the shift workers? It depends on what type of shifts we are dealing with. If we have to do a rare and one-off night shift, such as when babysitting for friends and waiting up for them to come home, or if doing a one-off overnight stock take, then it probably doesn't make sense to try to alter our body clock to fit in with this. It will have to be pulled and twisted back into its original shape the very next night. Instead, perhaps it is important here that we do what we can to cope with this one-off change, by napping earlier in the day and by increasing our alertness with caffeine, for example.

If, however, we just got a job as a nightclub bouncer and know that we will be up at night for the foreseeable future, it makes sense to shift our rhythm to cope with our new schedule as soon as we can. For example, the times we are exposed to light and dark, and when we choose to eat, drink and sleep, will be giving our bodies important cues about when to behave in specific ways. But it's not always that simple, as it's impossible to change the world around us – and regardless of what we do, the natural light and dark in our surroundings will send confusing messages to shift workers. There are drugs that can be used to aid rest, such as melatonin, and those that can facilitate alertness, such as modafinil. But drugs do not come risk-free and should never be taken without serious consideration from a doctor. Finally, perhaps those of us who are most likely to be vulnerable to physical and mental health disorders should consider whether it is possible to abstain from shift work entirely. If not, it might be worth checking health regularly.

Not long ago people could smoke on flights, in offices and pubs, putting the health of others at risk. This seems ridiculous now, yet we are still expected to work long hours, and handle stressful jobs and schedules that might increase our risk of certain problems. Future changes will surely aim to improve the sleep of the workforce and to protect our many vital shift workers. But will there be a day when long hours and shift work are a thing of the past? When I think of desperate phone calls for ambulances in the depth of the night – I am so grateful for the rapid help from telephone operators, first responders, paramedics and hospital staff, especially when they are putting their own health on the line to be there.

Pushing 40 and still no sleep

Middle-adulthood is sometimes described as the rush-hour years of our lives. We might be striving to make romantic relationships work, and our responsibilities can increase as we care for those both older and younger than us. Most people need to work too in order to make life financially viable. The stresses involved in all of this can leave us sleepless. At this stage in life, we often have to give our time over to others and we put ourselves second or even third. Perhaps we need to take advice from that glossy magazine and make sure we find some 'me time'. And if we manage, for the sake of our relationships and our careers, it might not be a bad idea to spend it fast asleep.

CHAPTER EIGHT

It's a Long Hard Night:
The Sleep of Older Adults

Older adults (65+ years) recommended 7–8 hours of sleep per 24 hours[1]

Olive Cooke was an asset to society. Even in her 90s she could be found selling poppies ahead of Remembrance Day to raise money for injured servicemen and women.[2] Yet, it was reported in the press that on 6 May 2015, aged 92, her body was found at the bottom of a gorge – she had taken her own life. A suicide note for her family reported that her life had become unbearable. Among other difficulties, including depression and ill health, she was no longer able to sleep, getting very few hours a night – and she could take it no more.

Her story touched people all over Britain and the prime minister made a statement about her death. However, the inclusion of sleep among the issues that she flagged were relatable to many. Older adults so often suffer with their sleep and this can be excruciating. So what should be expected of sleep at this stage in life and why?

Senior sleep

Earlier we discussed a strange shift in sleep timing during adolescence. Bedtime moves to a later time and it becomes much harder to wake up early in the morning. Well, flip this over and you have the typical sleep of an older adult – it's hard to stay up late and bedtime moves earlier. If our grandparents are first to leave the party, we now know why. These differences between us might make good evolutionary sense – if there is always someone awake and able to watch over the group, we're more likely to stay safe.[3] This has been referred to as the 'poorly

sleeping grandparent' hypothesis – older group members are
up early or sleepless at night and will watch over the others.
The hope is that the patterns of sleep in younger people will
allow them to repay the favour – so there is always someone
who is awake. Data supports this idea, and a study was carried
out by researchers from Canada, the USA and Tanzania,
examining sleep patterns in the Hadza hunter-gatherers from
the latter country. The Hadza typically live in groups of
around 30 people. Men tend to take the lead in hunting for
food such as birds and honey, and women are more likely to
lead the gathering of foods including nuts, seeds and fruits.
Hunter-gatherers are sometimes studied in the hope that they
will provide information about how people, who no longer
live in this way, might have existed in the distant past.* In this
study, it was found that during the 20 days in which the
group – whose participating members varied in age from 18
years upwards – was studied, there was only an 18-minute
period in which all members were asleep at the same time.
That meant that at any one time, someone was almost always
awake and able to keep an eye on what was happening in the
surrounding world. When we are asleep we lack vigilance and
are vulnerable so it is useful to have a night watchman.

Sleep stages change over time too and as we enter the golden
years of our lives we experience lighter sleep.[4] But with
increasingly light sleep comes an inevitable decrease in the
other stages. We get less REM and deep, slow-wave sleep. It
has been proposed that a reduction in slow-wave sleep – which
is important for our physical and mental restoration – could
even signify an age-related deterioration of the central nervous
system.[5]

Certain disturbances and problems with our slumber spike
at this stage of life and as we age we typically spend a greater
proportion of the night awake[4] – perhaps lying in bed with
just our thoughts. Sleep apnoea and restless legs syndrome are
common in older adults too.[6]

---

* This approach is imperfect as conclusions can differ depending on
the specific group under investigation.

When I talk to Marco, a retired university lecturer aged 79, about his sleep patterns, he tells me: 'I prefer to go to bed around 10 p.m. I never wake fewer than three times – to urinate – before sleep ends around 5.30 a.m. The longest time I sleep is three hours, although I had a single record-breaking four-hour phase a few months ago.' When I ask him how this relates to his peers, he tells me that he rarely discusses his sleep with them, but on the odd occasion that he does they nod knowingly as if members of a secret club.

Marco's situation is more extreme than many others of his age, but there are data to back up some of his experiences. Going to urinate during the night (known as nocturia) may become more frequent in older adults, and when it occurs regularly, it can be a key factor in disturbing sleep.[7] It is also very common, with around 80 per cent of those at Marco's stage of life going to the toilet at least once during the night.[8] However, multiple trips to the toilet are less common. If that does occur it can be worth investigating why this is happening, in case intervention is needed. Causes can vary but might include the body increasing urine production at night, depression leading to night wakings or a sleep disorder such as sleep apnoea waking the sufferer. All in all, when older relatives complain about their sleep, they probably have every right to do so.

Just consider the magnitude of the problem. It has been projected that in England by 2020 almost half of the adult population will be over 50 years of age.[9] And a large proportion of these will report a regular sleep problem. This suggestion is in line with a study of over 9,000 older adults, of whom more than 50 per cent reported a regular sleep complaint.[10] All this means that a lot of our friends, neighbours and loved ones are sleepy during the day, or lying awake in the still of the night, perhaps feeling miserable about their sleep.

Why do these changes occur?

It is likely that lots of things are going on to bring about these sleep changes and problems. The ageing process results in alterations in our brain, some of which may affect our sleep. As discussed in Chapter 1, sleep is brought about by a complex dance between different areas of the brain vying to turn each other on and off in order to bring about sleep and wakefulness. Death of neurons in brain areas such as the ventrolateral preoptic (VLPO) nucleus of the hypothalamus in older adults, an area centrally important in bringing about sleep, could therefore lead to problems when hitting the hay.[11]

Behavioural changes

Changes in behaviour are also likely to lead to problems. Of course, the behaviour of many older adults is far from stereotypical and we live in a colourful society where youths set up multi-billion-dollar businesses from their bedrooms and centenarians run marathons. However, there are also more stereotypical trends that may help to explain certain sleep changes. These include spending more time at home or, for some, in care homes. With that might come reduced exercise and exposure to light, coupled with increased opportunities for napping.

Spending long periods of time at home, and not seeing friends, family and neighbours, could result in poor-quality relationships. This could in turn lead to loneliness – a complaint that is common in older adults.[12] Loneliness – something we have all felt at some point – involves feeling that our social network is not up to scratch, which can reduce feelings of safety.[13] Feeling safe is important when it comes to our sleep, as it's unwise to lose consciousness if we think that harm might come to us, so perhaps it is perceived vulnerability that links loneliness and poor sleep quality. Our sleep becomes fragmented, allowing us to stay alert to danger. Loneliness can be particularly pronounced in older adults once they retire from their jobs, lose friends and become frailer. But of course loneliness is not a problem unique to older adults. I collaborated on a study led by researchers at King's College London, investigating sleep quality and loneliness in young adults. We found that those who reported feeling lonely also reported poorer sleep quality, with associated problems during the day.[14] Sadly, this relationship was particularly strong in those who had been exposed to violence or maltreatment in the past. Perhaps this was because they were more likely to see the world in which they live as a dangerous and threatening place. Maybe these people were more likely to stay awake because they felt that nobody had their back or because the abuse they had experienced in the past had occurred at night. Improving social networks, whether through more time spent with friends, engaging in local activities or attending adult courses, could be one route to reducing loneliness and benefitting sleep.

Hormonal changes

Age-related changes in behaviour may influence sleep, but alterations in behaviour do not explain all of the sleep changes experienced in older adults. How do they account for poor sleep experienced by the 'glammy grannies' who are members of tennis clubs and are drowning in friends and social activities? They could teach people half their age a thing or two about getting exercise, exposure to sunlight and living life to the full, yet some still struggle terribly with their sleep. So, which aspects of ageing, other than lifestyle, might explain these sleep alterations?

Hormonal changes are one possibility, especially in women. Women's oestrogen and progesterone levels plummet during menopause, which usually occurs earlier in adulthood, at around the age of 50. It can lead to symptoms such as hot flushes, anxiety and depression – and all these things can seriously impair a good night's sleep.

Marco, the retired university lecturer, suggests that I talk to his wife Maria, a sculptor, about her sleep. She has recently turned 75 and describes her menopause affecting her sleep in a way that seems to chime well with reports from others.[15] She tells me: 'I first suspected I was undergoing menopause when my periods started getting lighter I felt more anxious than usual and found my sleep became more and more disturbed. My joints felt more painful and particularly so at night. I would wake up feeling intense heat around my face and neck. I felt trapped in the burning furnace of my body. Nothing would cool it. Even in the coldest of nights I threw off all my covers and still felt internally hot, though aware that my feet were freezing. My sister-in-law was experiencing the same thing at around the same time and described having to change sheets at night as they were drenched with her sweat.'

Exploring this topic, a study of women aged 40–59 focused on self-reported sleep duration and quality in relation to menopausal status.[16] Whereas just 33 per cent of premenopausal women claimed to sleep for fewer than seven hours a night, this was 41 per cent in postmenopausal women. A greater proportion still (56 per cent) of women in a transition stage called perimenopause reported sleeping for less than seven hours a night.

Postmenopausal women were also more likely to report sleep problems and to wake up feeling unrefreshed compared with the premenopausal women. Maria's description is in line with the research findings and she ends by telling me: 'I have never managed to regain my good sleeping habits. Sleep has become something I do reluctantly. The pleasure of sleep is something of the past.'

Health and the ageing body

Physical ailments are also linked to sleep quality and may clock up over the course of one's life, or appear at a greater rate as we age. Cancer, diabetes, Alzheimer's, Parkinson's and enlarged prostate are just a few of the problems that are more common as we grow older – and have been linked to poorer sleep. The mechanisms linking these problems to sleep are diverse – and discussed later in this chapter – but pain and discomfort, toilet trips during the night, as well as the impact of certain medications taken for these ailments, are just some of the routes by which physical illness can disrupt our sleep.

Visual impairment

Our entire bodies suffer with the ageing process. However, as discussed by Professors Steven Lockley and Russell Foster, one particularly interesting change concerns the eyes, which begin to yellow. It's not that our eyes start to resemble those of an owl, but rather that the lenses of our eyes yellow.[17] This is caused by a build-up of pigment over time and reduces the amount of blue light that is passed to our retinas. It's even been suggested that older artists use more blue paint in their work for this very reason.[18] Changes to the eyes provides one fascinating route by which the ageing process may be linked to sleep, as it is this same blue light that is most significant in setting our body clocks and can prevent our bodies from making the darkness hormone melatonin when we look at our tablet or phone late at night. So, with a newly formed blue light filter in our eyes, the light cues around us might become less useful in influencing sleep timing. This could help to explain why older adults may go to bed earlier than others. But, be warned – this shouldn't be an excuse for older adults to use tablets last thing at night, as sleep hygiene remains important at this time of life when insomnia and other complaints are common.

Other eye-related changes during ageing can also potentially disturb sleep. One example is the clouding of the lenses known as cataracts, which limits the amount of light passed on to the retina of the eye. Cataract surgery involves swapping the cloudy lens for a clear one, so is perhaps not for the faint hearted. However, the advantages of getting cataracts sorted could potentially go beyond just improving vision, to help improve sleep too.[19]

Cataracts are a leading cause of blindness, but there are many other causes. The links between sleep and visual impairment are dramatic. Author of the book *Patient H69*, Vanessa Potter, was aged 41 and juggling a busy job and kids when she became blind after a rare neurological illness. She describes in her book how it became difficult to sleep once her illness set in. It distressed her to the extent that she made a 'deal with the devil' that if she were permitted to sleep again she would accept permanent blindness.[20] A few years on, Potter has relearned to see and her sleep has returned to normal.

Over half of those whose eyes are not able to detect any light at all suffer from a non-24-hour sleep–wake rhythm disorder, also known as free-running disorder. Here the master body clock strikes out of time with the world around us. For most people, the natural day is longer than 24 hours, so without light to keep the body clock in check, we might go to sleep progressively later each night, becoming out of sync with our environment. This can accumulate quickly, and if the time we go to sleep gets 30 minutes later each night, our 10 p.m. journey to the land of nod on a Monday could turn into a 1 a.m. bedtime by Sunday. Imagine how difficult this would be to live with when work requires us to get up first thing in the morning and we end up feeling groggy during the day. Fortunately, for most of us, light and other cues stop bedtime from creeping back in this way, but where this does occur, there is help at hand and carefully timed melatonin, for example, can help to treat this disorder.[21]

Interestingly, even in some people who are considered to be totally blind, the eyes can detect light via a relatively recently discovered mechanism. It turned out that in addition to the 'rods and cones' that help us see, which we learnt about in biology classes at school, there are other cells in the eye that detect light. These cells, called 'photosensitive retinal ganglion cells', send messages to the brain and help the master clock to lock onto the external environment. This means that as with their sighted peers, some people who are otherwise totally blind may benefit from exposure to light in the morning and darkness in the evening to help sync their body with the world around them.[17] Doctors sometimes recommend removing the eyes of those who have no sight for reasons such as when the eyeball is badly damaged. This decision is of course a big one, and doing so can cause sleep problems in those who are still able to detect light and use it to help set their body clocks regardless of their blindness.[17]

Mental health

Despite the challenges of ageing, older adulthood can be joyous. It can be a time to seize opportunities that life has so far prevented us from taking, whether studying art, music, literature or even learning to dive. Grandparents can also spend quality time with their grandchildren, time they simply did not have when raising their own children. Would it be going too far to suggest that retirement might allow us time to live in an orderly home, and to wake up to the smell of freshly baked croissants and a newspaper? This is my own fantasy, but this period of life can also bring psychological challenges. Dealing with our own mortality, or that of loved ones, can come at a huge psychological cost.

Stressful life events can contribute to the development of anxiety and depression and then, for some, there is the loss of a partner and a warm bed turns cold. Sleep disruption caused by tussles for the duvet gives way to that due to a newfound stillness at night. Perhaps unsurprisingly, scientific research shows that older adults who are grieving experience less sleep, and that which they do get is of a poorer quality compared with others – an association mainly explained by feeling depressed.[22]

Stress may also result in certain thought processes that are not conducive to a good night's sleep. The relationship between thoughts and the way in which older adults sleep is a topic that I investigated some years back. Together with an excellent team, including the undergraduate student Sophie Yearall and a post-doctoral researcher, Tom Willis, I wanted to examine sleep-related thoughts in older adults. In particular, we wanted to learn more about topics that may keep people awake at night. Yearall made visits to a local community hall and sheltered housing accommodation in south London, where she asked older adults about their thoughts concerning sleep in general and also specifically in the period before they fell asleep.[23] As had been found in the past among younger participants, in our study poorer sleep quality was associated with more dysfunctional beliefs about sleep – such as needing to try harder when not being able to sleep. There was also a link between feeling wound up before bedtime, and catastrophising about the consequences of not sleeping and sleeping poorly. Concerns that worried our participants when they could not sleep showed some differences to those raised by participants at other stages of life. For example, there were concerns about clumsiness, routine disruption, physical health or needing to take more medication. Family and social concerns, such as becoming socially isolated, were also expressed. Such findings support the idea that when addressing sleep problems, it is important to consider the way that older adults are thinking and to appreciate that people will have different concerns related to their sleep at different stages of their lives. Help provided needs to be tailored accordingly.

So, it seems that there are multiple reasons why sleep can become disrupted as we age – but which risk factors are most salient? A review study published in 2016 compared risk factors. It was found that rather than age itself, the greatest predictors of poor sleep in older adulthood were being female, feeling depressed and being physically unwell.[24] Older people falling into these categories might particularly need support to help them sleep well.

How do sleep problems marry up with performance and health as we age?

Given that poor sleep has been linked to so many challenges throughout life, should we worry about what our sleep-deprived elderly population may have waiting for them? Well, to start with the good news, it seems that older adults might be better at tolerating sleep deprivation than younger adults. In one study, older (aged 65–76) and younger (aged 18–29) adults were kept awake for 26 hours.[25] During this time they were regularly asked to report on their own sleepiness and were also given a task every other hour, which assessed their reaction time over a 10-minute period. Compared with the younger adults, the older ones seemed to experience fewer problems as the sleep deprivation progressed. At the outset, participants in both age groups performed well, but after 16 hours the younger participants began to flag whereas the older ones had fewer lapses in their performance and fewer attention failures. Despite this positive message, not all experts agree with the conclusion that older adults are better than others at tolerating lost sleep. It is also clear that poor sleep and sleeplessness is not good at any stage of life – and might not help with the ageing process.

Take short sleep and that of poor quality, for example. A number of studies have looked at these things in relation to telomere length.[26] Telomeres are structures at the end of our chromosomes that provide them with protection (a bit like wearing a hard hat on a building site). They shorten as our bodies age. Short telomeres are also linked to a plethora of health problems such as cardiovascular disease, obesity and depression. In various studies, although with mixed results, it has been found that those who miss out on sleep or report poor sleep quality tend to have shorter white blood cell telomeres than others. This is not only true of adults, but has even been reported in children.[27] While the mechanisms underlying these associations still need to be unravelled, this provides novel understanding of one way in which sleep length and quality could be linked to ageing.

Cognitive problems

Another way in which sleep may be linked to the ageing process is via reduced cognitive performance in older adults. It's not that we receive our free bus pass and suddenly become less smart. Just Google the age at which people have become Nobel Laureates in recent years and we can see the average age is 66 – and older in certain categories, such as literature, where the average age is 72.[28]

However, in some cases, cognitive problems do develop over time, and in a meta-analysis of studies of older adults addressing sleep length and cognition, it was found that those who reported short sleep and – interestingly – long sleep had poorer mental function in lots of different areas.[29] They included problems with executive function, memory of words, and the ability to hold information in a way that allows us to manipulate it to make decisions and guide behaviour. Just like Goldilocks and her porridge, extremes proved problematic. Why might this be? There are lots of possible explanations. The link with short sleep may seem obvious given the emphasis throughout this book on the importance of sleep. For example, not getting enough sleep could mean that the toxic protein beta amyloid, so central in the development of Alzheimer's, is not being properly cleared from the brain, leading to cognitive difficulties. The link with long sleep is less intuitive. Surely getting a lengthy kip is a good thing? But long sleep is associated with multiple different problems. One explanation is that long sleep could lead to a disruption of our biological rhythm. Just as those who sleep for short periods or at the wrong times may be forced to stay awake when their body is better suited to sleeping, so perhaps long sleepers are snoozing when their bodies are screaming at them to be awake. Long sleep could also lead to poorer sleep quality overall. Change your bedtime from 11 p.m. to 9 p.m. and you'll see what I mean – sleep becomes less efficient. Long sleep could also be a sign of mental and physical health problems that occur alongside other difficulties, and these links too might help to explain why long sleep is sometimes associated with negative outcomes.

Neurodegenerative disorders

Sleep changes are often a central feature of neurodegenerative disorders such as Alzheimer's disease. This disease touches so many. One of my earliest childhood memories is of visiting my great-granny Betty – who had Alzheimer's – in a nursing home. Regardless of the time of day we visited, she was often dozing when we arrived and was always forgetful and confused. She would wander off given half a chance and I'm not sure she knew who any of us were. Regardless, she retained some of the joy she'd had during her youth and would occasionally emit a resounding chortle.

Granny Betty's behaviour in her later years reflected her condition, which involved a change in certain brain functions, perhaps most notably memory. Sleep disturbances can be a risk factor for developing Alzheimer's – and may even occur prior to the cognitive decline characteristic of this disease. Once Alzheimer's sets in a patient may suffer from excessive daytime sleepiness and insomnia. There are also changes in sleep architecture, such as decreased amounts of REM and deep sleep.[30] All these problems appear to worsen with the severity of Alzheimer's and by the time the disease has fully set in a sufferer may be unable to sleep well at night. Instead they may sleep for short periods around the clock. In fact, it is often for this reason that loved ones are no longer able to look after someone with this condition, as there is no respite of a night's sleep. Instead, patients are sometimes cared for in nursing homes.

Parkinson's is another neurodegenerative disorder charac-terised by sleep anomalies. Someone with this disease will experience involuntary shaking of certain parts of the body, slow movement and stiff muscles. This disorder is discussed here in the older adult section of this book as its occurrence increases with age. However, as with other difficulties discussed here, this may also occur earlier in life. Notable examples include Michael J. Fox, 1980s Hollywood legend and teen heart-throb, who was diagnosed with this disorder in his 30s; as well as the boxer and activist Muhammad Ali, who was diagnosed in his 40s. The sleep disturbances seen in Parkinson's patients vary in type and often begin before they are diagnosed with the condition. They may include insomnia, restless legs syndrome and daytime sleepiness.[31]

Perhaps the most striking example of a sleep disorder seen in Parkinson's patients is REM sleep behaviour disorder. This rare disorder occurs when the usual paralysis accompanying REM sleep stops working. In some ways, it's the opposite of sleep paralysis. Instead of the paralysis from REM sleep continuing into our waking lives, our ability to move is carried over into REM sleep. Dreams are acted out – perhaps with complex motor behaviours or vocalisations. Episodes might involve lashing out, yelling or swearing in response to a dreamed threat. Less frequently, actions are non-violent, perhaps involving dancing, laughing or singing. Eyes can be shut the whole time. At the end of an episode, the sufferer might wake up and be quite coherent – able to recall the dream that elicited the actions of the night. This is different from other sleep disorders discussed earlier in this book – such as night terrors, which occur during deep sleep. What is concerning about this specific disorder is that it seems so strongly to predict the development of Parkinson's disease or other disorders. In fact, in one study, 29 men who had been diagnosed with REM sleep behaviour disorder were followed up over many years.[32] Dramatically, around 80 per cent of them went on to develop Parkinson's disease or dementia. This sounds alarming, but it's noteworthy that this study focused on men over 50 years of age and for whom it was unclear why they had this sleep disorder. In other words, the REM sleep behaviour disorder was idiopathic, meaning it could not be explained as a symptom of something else, such as a head injury or a psychiatric disorder. We wouldn't necessarily expect this dramatic association in a younger population, who are more likely to experience REM sleep behaviour disorder for other reasons – such as in response to certain medications for depression or because they are suffering from post-traumatic stress disorder. So, if you are showing signs of this sleep disorder, don't panic, but rather talk to your doctor to try to understand what is going on.

As to why sleep and neurodegenerative disorders might be linked, multiple mechanisms have been proposed.[33] Historically, sleep problems have been considered a consequence of these disorders. For example, Parkinson's can cause sleep problems because of changes to brain structures and neurotransmitters involved in sleep, as well as pain, or the drugs used to treat this disorder. However, turning this on its head, it is now believed that sleep problems also play a role in the development of neurodegenerative disorders. Perhaps the most well-established association is the aforementioned link between sleep and the build-up of beta amyloid amino acids in the brain, which is a key feature of Alzheimer's disease. It's not that lack of sleep is causing the accumulation of beta amyloid amino acids, but rather that without sleep they are not being cleared so efficiently from the brain.[33] There are multiple other possible mechanisms linking sleep and brain degeneration, such as a lack of sleep resulting in inflammation in the brain, which could then put the brain at risk of decline. With an absence of evidence, many hypotheses about why we find these associations remain little more than speculation.

Considering the links between sleep and neurodegenerative disorders provides me with a moment to appreciate my health while it lasts and to acknowledge the multiple challenges faced by sufferers of these disorders. It also provides a possible route by which to help.[33] Carefully timed exposure to bright light, information about sleep hygiene, cognitive behavioural therapy for treating insomnia, as well as, in some cases, medications for sleep problems, all hold promise for improving both daytime and nighttime for sufferers of some currently incurable diseases.

Cardiovascular outcomes and diabetes

Earlier in this book (see Chapter 6), a link between sleep and weight was discussed. It was also pointed out that shift work increases the risk of heart attacks and strokes. It should therefore perhaps come as no surprise that other aspects of our sleep have also been linked to issues such as diabetes, strokes and heart attacks. The amount of time that we spend sleeping can influence our insulin sensitivity and glucose tolerance, providing one way in which sleep is linked to the development of diabetes.[34] Diabetes is a risk for diseases affecting the heart and blood vessels too, which might also provide one of many possible explanations for the link between sleep length and cardiovascular outcome.[35] Short sleep can also lead to the silent build-up of calcium in the heart, providing another mechanism by which it increases risk of a cardiac event.[36] Sleep apnoea is also associated with cardiovascular events,[37,38] in part because a lack of oxygen in the blood can increase its pressure. This is because the body is doing what it can to compensate for low levels of oxygen, by increasing blood pressure to ensure that the vital organs get the oxygen they need at a time of limited supply.

Cancer

Then there is cancer, which is yet another devastating disease. In addition to the concerning links with shift work discussed previously, other aspects of our sleep may also be linked to the development and progression of this condition. There have been hypothesised links between short sleep, long sleep, naps, poor sleep quality and cancer. Reviewing experimental and epidemiological studies looking at more than 1.5 million participants from 13 countries, a group of scientists attempted to understand the relationship between sleep and cancer.[39] They concluded that experimental data and proposed mechanisms were consistent with the idea that certain aspects of our sleep could lead to cancer. By contrast, when they examined this association outside of the laboratory, looking at epidemiological data, the picture was far murkier and clear conclusions could not be drawn. This is not to say that associations do not exist in the real world, but rather that future studies need to consider the potential links between sleep and cancer more systematically before strong conclusions can be drawn.

Another feature of sleep linked to cancer is sleep-disordered breathing, where we repeatedly stop breathing for periods during the night or where breathing becomes shallow and we are not taking in enough oxygen.[40] In a study by scientists from the USA and Spain, sleep-disordered breathing was assessed in the sleep laboratory.[41] Participants were categorised by the existence and severity of their breathing problems. The participants were then followed for up to 22 years, and the authors looked to see whether there was a link between sleep-disordered breathing at that first assessment and subsequent deaths from cancer. There was a clear dose-response relationship, meaning that the greater the breathing problems as assessed in the laboratory, the bigger the chance of dying from cancer later in life. This link may seem surprising, but perhaps makes more sense when we look at animal studies, with a study of mice showing a worrying link between hypoxia (or oxygen deprivation) and the growth of cancer tumours.[42] This provides yet another reminder never to ignore breathing problems at night.

Other health issues

The list of heinous disorders that have been associated with the way we sleep continues to grow. However, even when we move away from the most worrisome health issues and focus on day-to-day ailments such as the common cold, our sleep still appears relevant. Could it be that the way we sleep is linked to the amount of time we spend sneezing and blowing our noses during the pesky winter months? It would seem so.

In a study published in 2015, the sleep of 164 people was assessed over a week.[43] The participants were then given some nasal drops containing rhinovirus, a viral infection that can cause the common cold. They were followed for five days to see if they became ill. As assessed by actigraphs (watch-like devices), those who slept for short periods (up to six hours a night) were more likely to develop a cold than those who slept for longer periods (more than seven hours a night).* Perhaps this is because our immune system is compromised when we are sleep deprived. Even one night of missed sleep can increase inflammation, making our bodies respond as if they are fighting an infection.[44] Whatever the link, these results chime well with life experience. When we're run-down it sometimes feels that just one late night can tip us over the edge and send us to bed for a week.

---

* When sleep length was assessed by self-report this association was not found. Perhaps participants were not very good at estimating their sleep length? It is unclear as to why this was the case. In the field as a whole, researchers sometimes reach different conclusions in their work depending on the way in which sleep is assessed.

Sleeping on the ward

With really bad luck, the downward spiral of poor sleep and health can land us in hospital. That in itself can create havoc for our sleep.[45] Perhaps the medical profession misses a trick by not showing more respect for the sleep of patients. Wards are shared by chattering folk, and lights are often kept on around the clock. This is true not only for older adults but for patients at every stage of life.

Worse still, is it possible that experiences while hospitalised could have an enduring negative impact upon our sleep? Will young children who have been woken in a hospital emergency, with blood being taken or tubes inserted into their nostrils while still half asleep, be left unable to sleep as soundly once they are home as they did previously? After all, this might be a reasonable response from a child who no longer believes that it is safe to sleep deeply. Such hypotheses need to be rigorously tested, but some research is consistent with the possibility that hospitalisation is a risk for sleep problems, with a small study finding higher levels of insomnia three months after discharge from hospital compared with previously.[46] While sleep is not always prioritised in hospitals, doctors and nurses have a difficult balance to strike. Staff can be up against limited resources, and a patient's desire to shut their curtains and turn off the lights to sleep is important, but it does not trump a nurse's need to monitor patients for potential deteriorating health during the night. This is a difficult balance to strike.

Surely more can be done to help the sick recover, and prescribing the natural remedy of sleep is likely to help. With this in mind, it's always inspiring to hear of the multiple initiatives under way, such as adjusting sound, light and temperature and minimising visits during the night in order to improve the sleep of those in hospital.[47] Not only could doing so give the body the best chance of recovery, but it might allow an earlier discharge, freeing up beds. Sleep can also reduce the suffering of patients and research suggests that people can perceive pain as more severe when sleep deprived.[48] In fact, the magnitude of the impact of sleep deprivation on pain perception has even been equated to that of certain painkillers. Next time we are in mild pain, it might not be a bad idea to reach for our pyjamas rather than pills.

Chronotherapy

As well as improving the sleep of those under their care, another way that doctors might eventually improve the outcome for their patients is to pay more attention to their body clocks. These are essential for so many of our physiological processes, explaining why certain times of the day may be best for going to bed, waking up, eating, sitting an exam, or even running a race. What is more, the symptoms of many of the illnesses we experience seem to be controlled in a clock-like manner, with peptic ulcers causing most grief at night,[49] for example. Similarly, symptoms of cancer, allergies, asthma, arthritis and cardiovascular disease, to name just a few, can fluctuate following a circadian pattern. So perhaps it is unsurprising that our body clock also appears to be important in predicting the effectiveness of certain medicines – and the extent of their side-effects. Chronotherapy refers to a consideration of just this and involves adapting our medical treatment to be in tune with our circadian rhythms. The aim is to optimise outcome.

This is becoming a popular research field and it seems that, just as coffee is best enjoyed first thing in the morning, certain drugs might be most beneficial if taken at certain times too. There are now hundreds of studies investigating this issue. A study by scientists from Birmingham in the UK found that giving older adults the influenza vaccination in the morning appeared to be more effective, in terms of antibody response, than administering it later in the day.[50] This was not found for all strains of the virus, and the study was small, but such results provide an example of how this type of work might potentially provide a cost-free way of improving public health.

Thinking ahead, could it be that the time of day we are called in for chemotherapy is literally the difference between life and death? The timing of drug administration might be particularly important in cases where the symptoms of the disease being treated wax and wane over the course of the day and night, such as for the aforementioned night-bothering peptic ulcers. Fast-forward 50 years and it's possible that the field of medicine will be revolutionised, with personalised medication and chronotherapy improving treatment outcome and reducing side-effects. But even with these likely improvements over time, sometimes even the best possible care and most carefully planned treatment cannot help, and death can be staved off no longer. Our inner clock plays a role at this final moment of life and may help to explain the time at which we come to take our final breath.

I'll sleep when I'm dead

Intuitively, there seems to be a link between sleep and death. When the time comes, we put our beloved pets to sleep and watch our loved ones sleep their way out of this life. But do our sleeping habits at other stages of life predict death? The answer might be yes. In a study published in 2003, 185 healthy older adults, mainly aged 60–80 years of age, were assessed in a sleep lab.[51] They were then followed up over 4 to 19 years, during which time 66 had died. The authors noticed that a number of aspects of sleep were important in predicting who had died during this period. For example, even after taking into consideration the age of the adults, and other things such as their medical problems when they were first assessed, those who took more than half an hour to fall asleep were more likely to die, as were those who spent more time awake during the night. There were also interesting links with sleep stages, and those who spent a particularly low or high proportion of their sleep in REM were also more likely to die. Results such as these should not be considered conclusive until there are a sufficient number of other studies that support them. However, they add to what we already know about the links between different aspects of sleep and our immune system, cardiovascular health and cancer. The idea that our sleep quality could be linked with our mortality is important.

The association between sleep length and death has long fascinated researchers and has been the topic of multiple meta-analyses. These have concluded that both short and long sleep may put a person at risk of dying sooner than those who sleep for a normal length of time.[52,53] Recent reviews have backed up these findings, with one report suggesting that those who sleep for short periods, compared with normal sleepers, have a 12 per cent increased risk of mortality when followed up a year or more later.[54] What is more, there was a linear association, with progressively short sleep of six hours or less associated with increased risk.[54] Interestingly, a dose-response relationship has also been reported for long sleep and an increased risk of death when followed up one or more years later.[55] Discussing this with Professor Buysse (see Chapter 1), he tells me: 'The most fascinating thing about the sleep duration–mortality relationship is that we could potentially do something about it. Although sleep has biological determinants, it is also partly a voluntary behaviour. What we need to know next is whether helping short sleepers to sleep longer could have a positive effect on physiology, and whether that, in turn, could help with long-term health and even mortality risk. The long-sleep side of the equation is a little trickier. I'm not sure that having long sleepers reduce their sleep will be a good idea. But, at the very least, we can continue to investigate what it is that long sleep does to our bodies to have this apparently negative effect.'

In addition to the complex relationship between sleep length and death, it seems that these two things are intertwined in other ways and that our body clocks might even influence the time at which we die. According to one report, death caused by disease, such as heart disease, rather than by trauma, such as getting run over by a car, was most likely to occur in the morning (peaking at 8 a.m.) and to a lesser extent in the afternoon (peaking at 6 p.m.).[56] Interestingly, timing of death may depend on the cause of death – as the symptoms of different diseases peak at different times of the day.[57] When we look at risk periods for cardiovascular events it seems that the morning is most dangerous. This could be because of the physiological changes occurring during this time, such as a peak in the stress hormone cortisol and an increase in blood pressure, which can put stress on the body.

I'll sleep before I'm dead

As we approach our twilight years, our changing bodies and lives can make it hard for us to nod off. Hormonal shifts, cell death in brain regions controlling sleep and changes to our eyes can all mean that sleep becomes more elusive than before. The sleep we do get is lighter than it once was and our bodies march out of time with others in society – we turn in for the night and wake up earlier than we once did. In a cruel twist, poor sleep also forecasts problems linked to ageing, such as cognitive difficulties.

Yet, sleep at this stage of life is not all bad, and some people sleep very well. Others who report feeling overwhelmed during the busiest stages of their lives yearn for old age, when they are able to apply the brakes and enjoy a lie-in if they so choose. This portion of life is sometimes accompanied by fewer responsibilities and can allow us to banish the alarm clock as well as enjoy new opportunities during the daytime. While sleep problems are common in older adults, they are certainly not an inevitable part of ageing and help is at hand. The next chapter offers advice and tips for getting that all-important shut-eye. To make the most of our precious days on earth, we must get the best sleep that we possibly can.

A Ticket to the Land of Nod: Tips to Get Your Best Sleep and Make Dreams Come True

The sleep-deprivation epidemic?

Having arrived at the last chapter of this book, you should now be convinced that sleep matters. It is a pillar of health that is so often neglected and we need to make sure we embrace it if we are to be the best versions of ourselves. The assertion that we might want to prioritise our sleep may be coupled with the realisation that we are massively sleep deprived. Many achieve nothing like the seven to nine hours recommended for most adults.[1] This might be unsurprising to you given that the media so commonly declare there to be a sleep-deprivation epidemic.[2] But what does that really mean and is it *really* happening? Recent epidemics involve the Ebola virus and avian influenza (H7N9), also known as 'bird flu'. While not getting enough kip is clearly not an infectious disease, the term 'epidemic' might be used in this context to imply that sleep deprivation is widespread and the common nature of it is something new.

First, let's consider whether insufficient sleep really is widespread. Many of us clock up far fewer hours asleep than the recommended amount. This was flagged clearly in a 2012 survey of national health in the USA – which polled more than 300,000 adults[3] – where 29 per cent claimed to sleep for no more than six hours each night. The same is true of people at other stages of life and in the National Sleep Foundation's Sleep in America poll, almost half of the adolescents surveyed reported that on school nights they slept for fewer than the minimum recommended amount – eight hours.[4]

Whether this unsatisfactory situation is new is less clear. Many adults live in the fast lane, using caffeine to pull them through the day, and they might receive emails and calls late into the night. Others miss out on sleep by spending hours watching TV, playing video games or surfing the web. Some of these distractions would not have applied to our grandparents, who historically would not have had internet in their homes and might have spent more time reading good old-fashioned books or listening to the radio. But when we compare other aspects of our lives with those of our grandparents, did they really have more opportunity for slumber?

At the end of a day we can throw clothes into the washing machine and tumble dryer. If we want to, we can eat food, conveniently put together by someone else, which can take just seconds to prepare. Chicken can now be obtained from shops, pre-moulded into the shape of teddy bears to delight the children, and potatoes can come out of their wrappers mashed and rehashed exotically for our satisfaction. The dishwasher cleans our dishes and we can have a warm bath at the turn of a tap.

But what about our grandparents or their ancestors? Were their lives more of a doddle? Clothes were handwashed and dried using a mangle and hung up to dry. Dinners were prepared from scratch (no chicken teddy bears for children born in the first half of the twentieth century). Of course, there was no dishwasher or central heating and the luxury of a bath involved painstakingly decanting boiling water into a metal tub. Would this really have allowed for an earlier bedtime?

And what about when we look back further to consider the impact of industrialisation on sleep? A team of researchers examined the sleep patterns of those living in three different isolated hunter-gatherer/horticulturalist societies from Bolivia, Namibia and Tanzania.[5] Using actiwatches to measure sleep, they found that the people in these societies slept for around the same length of time (on average 6.4 hours) as those in industrialised societies. They also went to sleep some three or so hours after sunset. Again, these largely reflected the sleep patterns of those living in industrialised societies. Is it possible that industrialisation, having led us to attend to our emails rather than the land, has not led to such great changes in the way we sleep after all? Not all experts agree.

According to Malcolm von Schantz, professor of chrono-biology at the University of Surrey: 'Studies on communities that are on the cusp of electrification (both in South America and in Africa) consistently suggest that the result is a delay in sleep phase. It makes sense that availability of light and entertainment encourages people to stay up later.' He continues: 'But does it mean that they also sleep less? Horacio de la Iglesia and colleagues found that to be the case when comparing two communities in Argentina. But when we did a similar comparison in Mozambique, we found no difference in sleep duration. I suspect this illustrates the great plasticity of human sleep. Electrification causes people to sleep later and may cause them to sleep less – but it also makes a big difference how long they are able to sleep in for in the morning.'

Other studies, focusing on different time periods, have directly tested the idea that we are getting less sleep over time, with mixed results. Some studies have reported changes over recent decades (or longer time periods) in adults[6] and also children and adolescents.[7,8] Other studies and reviews of the literature in adults, including one that focused on objective measures of sleep duration over the past 50 years, do not indicate changes at all.[9] In work led by Dr Kristen Knutson, a biomedical anthropologist at the University of Chicago, time diaries from eight different studies conducted between 1975 and 2006 were examined. These are 24-hour diaries in which participants provide open-ended information about the timing and duration of all of their activities. Overall, there was not a great deal of support for the idea that short sleep had become a greater issue over recent years.[10] 'This was true in everyone combined,' Dr Knutson tells me. 'But the proportion of short sleepers did increase among full-time workers, suggesting that employment characteristics may have led to an increase in short sleepers.' She went on to explain that studies tend to consider sleep in isolation from other factors – although the consequences of insufficient sleep need to be considered in relation to time and place. She provides an example: 'If sleeping less than six hours does indeed increase appetite as experimental studies suggest, but you are physically active or have limited access to food, obesity is not necessarily the result. If we want to understand how sleep patterns affect health, we need to study these associations in the specific culture or environment in which they occur.' In terms of the trends over time, overall it seems that many of us need more kip than we are actually getting – but perhaps we always did. Life gets in the way. However, the consequences of short sleep might be quite different today than they were in days gone by.

Sleep length aside, has sleep changed in other ways over time? The historian Roger Ekirch believes so. During the 1980s he was researching *At Day's Close* – a book focusing on night-time before the Industrial Revolution.[11] He found that something surprising kept cropping up – mentions of two sleeps. Discussing this with Ekirch, he reports 'The first references to "first" and "second" sleep were found in legal depositions at the old Public Record Office on Chancery Lane and in travel accounts, poetry and other literature from the late Middle Ages to the late 1700s.' He goes on to note that later he discovered European authors in the nineteenth century (including Dickens and Tolstoy) had also referred to the 'first' and 'second' sleep. Researching this topic, it became increasingly clear that pre-industrialisation, we normally went to bed between 9 p.m. and 10 p.m. We would then wake up shortly after midnight for an hour or so before enjoying a second sleep. The interval of wakefulness could be spent making love, contemplating dreams and doing so much more. It is interesting to think that this pattern of sleep could provide those suffering from sleep maintenance insomnia with an alternative model to lying in bed awake and worrying. The message is that when insomnia creeps up on us, we shouldn't sweat it. Perhaps instead we should simply enjoy our first and second sleep, and embrace the patterns of our ancestors.

Despite this comforting message, not everyone agrees with this. For example, the aforementioned research, examining the sleep patterns of those living in three different isolated hunter-gatherer/horticulturalist societies from Bolivia, Namibia and Tanzania, found no robust evidence that people in these communities woke up for extended periods during the night.[5] From this, it was argued that the bimodal sleep pattern described by Ekirch is perhaps not our natural state after all. Nevertheless, it is difficult to understand why the first and second sleep was reported so widely in pre-industrial Europe as well as non-European countries.[12] More research is needed to reconcile these different, yet monumental, contributions to our understanding of sleep.

Top tips for a better night's sleep

Regardless of whether or not we are experiencing a novel epidemic of sleeplessness, it is clear that many of us are in need of more sleep and are keen to improve the quality of that which we do get. This elixir is something we want to buy into, despite the expense of a shorter day. So, how might we obtain it?

Address health problems

Health problems can interfere with sleep and so need to be addressed. These include problems that occur while we are awake relating to both physical and mental health. Just as lumps and bumps need to be taken seriously and resolved quickly, so do issues concerning our mental health. Health problems that can interfere with sleep include sleep disorders – such as sleep apnoea, which is all too common in gentlemen of a certain age. As discussed in Chapter 8, it is associated with a plethora of problems including strokes and heart attacks.[13] People with sleep apnoea often report memory and cognitive difficulties[14] and can be left feeling exhausted during the day, increasing the risk of car and work accidents.[15] Sleep apnoea is pretty common, however although these associations are well established they are perhaps less well publicised. Many were shocked to hear that sleep apnoea contributed to the death of Carrie Fisher, who was so cherished for her role as Princess/General Leia in Star Wars.[16] Sleep experts were less surprised, as this disorder can put immense pressure on the body. The importance of diagnosing this sleep disorder crops up again and again, and was highlighted in 2016 when a train crashed in New Jersey, resulting in over 100 casualties. While we might never know the extent of its significance, the train driver involved in the accident was later found to have undiagnosed sleep apnoea.[17] This disorder should never be ignored and anyone with symptoms would be wise to visit their doctor, get a second opinion if necessary or try to reach a specialist.

Avoid sleeping pills

Perhaps counter-intuitively, another tip for getting good sleep is to consider carefully whether sleeping pills can be avoided. Starting early in life, children are sometimes offered melatonin to help them sleep. This can be helpful when treating certain children who struggle to sleep, and it might be useful when behavioural techniques have been unsuccessful.[18] However, as discussed in Chapter 3, there is a dearth of studies examining the long-term outcomes of this drug in children, a concern that is repeatedly flagged.[19]

Sleeping pills, sometimes taken by adults with insomnia, are also problematic as they do not bring about 'normal' sleep and can only ever mask rather than address any underlying issues. We might want to think twice about taking prescription drugs (including benzodiazepines and Z-drugs), as well as those purchased over the counter (including antihistamines and herbal remedies), and certainly avoid those available illegally.

The American College of Physicians notes that sleeping pills for insomnia have been associated with some worrying issues such as dementia and fractures – which may occur due to falling because of grogginess – and should only ever be taken for short periods.[20] These pills might be prescribed to help a patient cope with a period of unrelenting sleeplessness, such as that following the death of a loved one.

However, the use of pills needs to be considered on a case-by-case basis and it would be unwise to stop taking prescribed drugs without expert advice. Certainly, for some sleep disorders such as narcolepsy it could be dangerous to do so without consulting a doctor. The advice given in a book can never trump that provided by a doctor following careful consideration of a patient's history. But perhaps make sure you engage in an informed discussion with a doctor about whether sleep-related pills are really the very best way forward. Realise that any reluctance on the doctor's part to prescribe these drugs is likely to be medically founded. A colleague described a patient with insomnia requesting 'a bucket o' pills' – perhaps without realising that this was unlikely to produce his desired outcome of long-term sound sleep.

Instead of taking pills for insomnia, cognitive behavioural therapy can help overcome long-term sleeplessness, both in children[21] and adults.[20] Given that sleep is associated with so many aspects of our well-being, it's worth investing the time.

Think twice about gimmicks and devices

We might also want to think carefully about the devices we buy in order to help us sleep. Sleep should be an automatic process and not one that is effortful or contrived. Oxford Professor Colin Espie (mentioned in Chapter 7) draws an amusing parallel between sleep, sex and golf. He points out that when we think about our performance in these things too much, it all goes dramatically wrong.

With that in mind, do we really need a teddy bear that emits sounds resembling the inner gurglings of the womb? And what about that rock music that has been vamped into lullabies? Or the autonomous sensory meridian response videos that aim to produce a tingling sensation primarily on the scalp and neck in response to visual and auditory stimuli, and could lead to relaxation that might just help us nod off? Can we live without the watch-like devices that we use to track our sleep, or the clamp designed to stop our partners nicking the bed sheets? And what about that hoodie that can double up as a cushion, or the 'boyfriend pillow' that allows us to sleep with an arm around us? Will that beautiful silk eye mask from an expensive store ever be worn? The number of commercial devices to help us sleep is growing all the time, but are they really helpful?

Some are well conceived and might indeed be useful, but it is also possible that some could disturb our sleep or we could become dependent on them to nod off. A colleague described how she became obsessed with her sleep after buying a device to track it. She was endlessly competitive with herself, and would will herself to beat her previous night's statistics in terms of the length and quality of her sleep. This did her no favours, and instead she ended up lying in bed wide awake.

Consider exercise and food

Exercise provides another useful way to help us sleep (see Chapter 6) and sun salutations in the park in the morning may bring the added benefit of light exposure first thing. When I spoke to Marco, the retired university lecturer, he told me that his sleep tends to be better the more physically active he has been during the day. Marco also mentions food and alcohol, which he says can disturb his sleep if taken after 7 p.m.

Thinking about what passes our lips can indeed be useful. Most of us will have been told at some point in our lives what to eat or drink in order to get a better night's sleep. We may have been told not to eat cheese before bedtime, as it will give us nightmares. Perhaps we've been encouraged to have a nightcap to help us nod off. Or should we replace coffee with a chamomile tea in order to help us relax at night? What about a lavender biscuit before bed? Should we change our online shopping basket based on these suggestions? Before clicking, it's worth considering the evidence.

To start with the pantomime villains of the world of sleep, perhaps the Captain Hook is caffeine.* A large

---

* Caffeine may be a problem for sleep, but it also has benefits such as reducing fatigue when required. It has also been used to successfully treat sleep apnoea in premature babies.[22]

proportion of adults drink coffee to help them wake up, which means that consumption before trying to sleep doesn't make a lot of sense. Of course, caffeine can be found in more than just coffee and tea. It's found in cocoa, chocolate, certain painkillers, green tea and some fizzy drinks too. We know that caffeine affects sleep, making it harder for us to nod off, and resulting in shorter, lighter and more disturbed sleep. We even understand the mechanism by which this works (remember adenosine from Chapter 1?).

People's sensitivity to caffeine differs greatly too – and the effect it has on sleep is influenced by age, sex, weight, as well as genetic differences between us.[23] Whereas some claim to be able to drink a vat of coffee before bedtime with seemingly no ill effects, others get jittery just at the thought. The former are able to experience the joys of a post-supper coffee, however they lose out on the benefits of using it to keep them awake when needed. As a general rule, we are advised to avoid caffeine as the day progresses. This is because it can hang around in our system for such a long time. An example of this comes from a study which found that consuming caffeine as many as six hours before bed can dramatically disrupt sleep.[24] Participants were given a dose of 400mg of caffeine, which is sometimes proposed to be around the safe daily limit for most adults, and which is more or less equivalent to four cups of home-brewed coffee or a very large one from your favourite coffee shop. The caffeine was taken either right before bed, or three or six hours beforehand. Even when participants went to bed six hours later, those that had consumed caffeine slept for around an hour less than those given a placebo. Taking this a step further, we might actually want to consider avoiding caffeine altogether, as it's been noted that it can stay in our bodies for such a long time that when consumed as early as 8 a.m. can result in more superficial sleep, even if we don't sink into bed until midnight.[23]

Then there is booze. Many of us reach for the bottle – be it wine, real ale or a G&T – after a gruelling day at work. The hope is that it will relax us and help us fall into a blissful slumber. It seems to do exactly that for a while. One mechanism behind this is that alcohol mimics the effects of GABA, first discussed in Chapter 1, which is a central neurotransmitter involved in helping us to get some shut-eye (and which you might remember is the focus of certain sleeping pills for insomnia). Consequently, when drinking alcohol we fall asleep more quickly and start the night resembling a log. There is less chance of waking and more time is spent in deeper sleep[25] – but that is where the good news ends. For example, one study found that when we look in detail at the 'deep sleep' experienced by those who have been drinking, it is a little unusual. It includes alpha brainwaves, which are more commonly seen when someone is awake and relaxing. This suggests that deep sleep following a night on the tiles might not be as restorative as it could be.[26] As for the second half of the night, it doesn't even pretend to be nice! During this time we are more likely to wake up and if we've drunk a lot we might miss out on REM sleep too.

Those who have slept next to someone who has had a skinful can likely attest that alcohol can increase snoring and the need for a tinkle during the night. When considering alcohol and sleep, perhaps most importantly we need to consider safety. Mixing alcohol and sleeping pills, for example, can be a lethal combination, as is so often and tragically reported in the press. All in all, when we consider the evidence, the offer of a nightcap becomes that bit less appealing.

The rest of what we know about the effects of our diet on our sleep is far less conclusive, although it seems that another baddy for our sleep could be a high-fat diet, which has been associated with problems including less sleep overall[27] and an increase in daytime sleepiness.[28] As the list of foods and drinks to avoid goes on, we might wonder whether it is best to just stop eating altogether! That's not the answer either, as severe calorie restriction can negatively affect our sleep.[29] Leah, a fitness enthusiast in her 20s, describes to me a period of her life when she was on the '5–2' diet, where she ate normally for five days a week and restricted her calorie intake to just 500 calories on the other two days. For the first time in her life she had real trouble sleeping. She exclaims: 'It was baffling because I usually sleep so easily and deeply.' So it would seem that restricting food can sometimes cause problems when trying to bunk down for the night, but what exactly should we be eating in order to sleep well?

If caffeine is the Captain Hook of foods when it comes to sleep, what is the Tinkerbell? Fatty fish perhaps? Tart cherry juice? This is not so clear cut, but numerous candidates are vying for the wand.[30] So what exactly are their claims to this accolade?

In a review of research focusing on how the foods that we consume are related to our sleep, a few groups were flagged as possibly beneficial.[30] Take a high-carbohydrate diet, for example. Although studies have provided an inconsistent picture, this might be associated with falling asleep more quickly (as well as increased REM sleep, although decreased slow-wave sleep). Foods containing high levels of carbohydrate include healthy foods such as vegetables and beans as well as less healthy ones such as cakes, chunks of fresh white bread and white pasta dishes. Some of these foods are those that the magazines tell us to avoid if we want to keep trim. But could it be that these very baddies might actually help us fall asleep?

Think back to our good friend melatonin via a circuitous route: when we consume carbohydrates, our bodies undergo changes, making the amino acid tryptophan more accessible to the brain. Tryptophan is a precursor of serotonin and melatonin. Does this mean that keeping a ready stash of biscuits by the bedside and scoffing them prior to sleep is the best way forward? Sadly not, as not only is the evidence to date weak, but the types of carbohydrates that we consume are likely to be important. Furthermore, the times at which we consume food need to be considered and we should eat at consistent and sensible times in order to maintain the synchrony of our internal circadian rhythms.[31]

Given the process by which high-carbohydrate foods can influence sleep, foods containing tryptophan directly – such as turkey, nuts, fish and milk – could potentially be useful in promoting our sleep. But here we come full-circle, as whether this tryptophan actually enters the brain depends somewhat on what else is going on in the body, such as the amount of carbohydrates consumed. As we were taught from the food guide pyramid in our home economics classes at school, foodstuffs should not be thought about in isolation, and future studies must further establish the food combinations and times at which we should eat in order to obtain optimal sleep. The psychological effects of food on sleep have also been proposed to be important – for example, it has been suggested that one route by which warm milk may encourage sleep is by eliciting childhood memories of bedtime rituals.[32]

Then there is food containing melatonin itself. Take tart cherry juice, for example. This may seem a somewhat unusual drink – and my guess is that most people won't have tasted it before – however, tart cherries (particularly Montmorency ones) are rich in melatonin.[33] One study found that consuming their juice resulted in higher levels of melatonin in urine samples and longer sleep of improved quality.[34] Human and animal melatonin levels are typically highest at night and for this reason it has been suggested that milk collected at this time may be particularly beneficial in promoting sleep.[32] The melatonin in cow's milk could make us feel sleepy, just as our mother's breast milk might have when we fed at night as a baby.

There is also a plethora of plants and herbs for which relaxing and sleep-promoting properties have been claimed. These include chamomile, kava and lemon balm.[35] The perennial plant valerian, which is typically consumed as a tea, has been given particular attention. Some sufferers of insomnia swear by it and there is also some support from certain studies that consumption leads to a perceived improvement in sleep. However, findings are inconsistent and there is little evidence that it has magical properties over placebo when sleep is measured objectively.[36]

Before we revamp our entire diet in an attempt to get better sleep and enjoy the associated benefits, we need to ask how much difference this will *really* make. Well, avoiding caffeine and alcohol can definitely be positive. As for what we should add to our diet, let's just say that I won't be making any changes to my shopping basket any time soon. Further work is needed in this area as the number of people included in studies is often small and results are inconsistent. We need to know more about food combinations and timings. Until we have this information, obtaining a healthy diet remains the best advice that we can receive – although, if dubious sleep benefits are used as a poor excuse to indulge in a bad diet from time to time, so be it.

Snooze and lose? Think hard about naps

Naps can be good for us, but might they also be bad? All of us have engaged in napping at some point in our lives. Certainly as infants and young children, but also often during times of physical stress such as pregnancy, illness and in the later stages of life. Napping instead of driving tired is always the better thing to do. A nap can leave us refreshed, alert and better able to function during the day. It can support our immune system, reduce our stress levels and sensitivity to pain and aid our mental well-being.[37] A snooze may be particularly powerful post lunch, when we experience a natural dip in our alertness and performance. Some swear by the 'nappucino', where we down a coffee and move rapidly on to a kip before the caffeine kicks in. The idea is we wake up raring to go.

Despite advantages, naps also have a dark side. A post-lunch rest can give us the kick we need to finish that overdue report or impress with our effervescent conversation – however, naps can also lead to sleep inertia, a groggy state. While we are often recommended to take short naps (of no longer than 20 minutes) to avoid this sleep inertia, even brief naps can sometimes lead to this undesirable state.[38] Napping can also leave our night-time sleep somewhat lacking. If we think back to Captain Obvious, the longer we are awake, the greater our sleep drive. If we've had a nap in the afternoon, the drive for sleep in the evening is reduced, which can make it harder to nod off. Marco, the retired lecturer, tells me this is certainly true in his case. This also appears to be a particular problem for those experiencing sleep disorders such as insomnia, which is why sufferers are typically told to avoid naps.

When it comes to naps, one size does not fit all. This was illustrated by a colleague who having read the research on naps, was convinced that she could benefit too. She even managed to persuade her husband to join her. Together they would crawl into bed at 1 p.m. each day. They would lie, side by side, willing themselves to fall asleep. Instead, they would end up staring blankly at the ceiling for a full 20 minutes before resuming their working day. After doing this for a week, they admitted defeat and concluded that while naps can be a good thing, they are certainly not for everyone.

Make love not war

Stress is one of the greatest poisons of our sleep, but sadly it's all around us. If we think about how we feel when stressed, perhaps when there is an exam coming up, when we have been shouted at by a teacher or boss, or are sitting in a traffic jam when we have somewhere to be, the effects on sleep will come as no surprise. In these situations our stress hormone cortisol increases, as does our adrenaline. Cortisol is usually low before bedtime and surges in the morning after we wake up. Intuitively, it would seem that a double shot of cortisol, served up without sugar and milk last thing at night, can't be a good thing. Adrenaline is the hormone that puts us in fight-or-flight mode – but do we really need to be ready for combat or to run away when we are simply trying to unwind before bed? Experimental data corroborates the idea that stress, such as being treated poorly by others, can result in difficulties nodding off.[39] Late at night our problem-solving skills are unlikely to be at their best and our sleep won't thank us for attempting to resolve issues at this time. What is more, mental and physical arousal before bed can prevent us sleeping. Instead, it might be worth trying to address any problems that we have well before bedtime. Heated discussions at night are best avoided.

And what about sex? Does a bit of intimacy help us to sleep well? Intuitively, yes. But there seems to be remarkably little research focusing on this. However, it does make sense that making love could lead to a better night's sleep, as a reason sometimes given for having sex in the first place is to reduce stress[40] and relaxation can increase post orgasm too.[41] Surely that is a good thing for sleep. This fits well with the mantra of the sleep expert that the bedroom should be reserved for sleep and sex only, perhaps implicitly emphasising that the latter is no bad thing when it comes to our slumber.

Avoid action in the bedroom

So, with permission to have sex in our bedrooms, is everything else really a no-no? Well, for those struggling with their sleep, that may very well be the case. Take reading books, for example. This antiquated bedtime ritual may do no harm to those who sleep easily and might well be among their greatest pleasures. However, for those struggling to nod off, it could lead to arousal.

And what about a bit of music before bed? Again, we might consider limiting this in the bedroom if we are struggling to sleep, although it's also noteworthy that listening to relaxing music can help to improve sleep in those who struggle with their slumber.[42] I contacted Kira Vibe Jespersen, author of the prestigious Cochrane Review* on listening to music for improving sleep in adults with insomnia, for her thoughts on this topic. She told me: 'There is some evidence to suggest that listening to music can improve subjective sleep quality in persons with sleep problems. This subjective effect of music on sleep is really important, but in terms of objective measures of sleep quality, we still need better quality studies to determine whether music can be helpful for this group.' In other words, listening to music might make us feel that we

---

* Cochrane Reviews provide a high standard of evidence-based information about healthcare.

have better quality sleep, but there is not yet much evidence from sleep labs to support this.

How does our sleep fare when it comes to other activities in the bedroom? Eggs Florentine in bed and other niceties can earn us adoration from our partners, and may be a one-off treat, but again aren't necessarily recommended for those struggling to sleep. Nor is working on assignments on the laptop in bed, or streaming movies and playing games.

So why aren't those with sleep difficulties allowed to have any fun? Why are they advised that they should restrict their bedroom activities to sex and sleep? Whereas reading, listening to music, eating and writing in bed may all be fine and even pleasant for those who consider themselves to be good sleepers, they also have the potential to be problematic in certain cases as they can reinforce the association between the bedroom and being awake. Clinicians describe how reading a book, watching a film, listening to music and other activities can be quite soporific for the majority, yet these same activities can sometimes cause real problems for those who are suffering from insomnia, reinforcing the problem. Perhaps the best advice is that if we want to read *War and Peace*, listen to Meatloaf or wolf down breakfast, we should find a suitable place to do so – and that might not be the bedroom.

Lack spontaneity

The excitement of a surprise visit to Rome might help to keep even the most quarrelsome of couples happy, however when it comes to a good night's sleep, a better approach might be to lack spontaneity and stick with what we know. We should do everything in the same way, at the same time, every day. Boring as it may sound, this is likely to do wonders for our sleep. When it comes to slumber, the more boring the better. A life of monotony is what we need! If we do the same thing every day, and have a consistent bedtime, our bodies learn that certain cues are associated with sleep. Our body naturally eases towards falling asleep at the same time each day. A consistent wake time is important too and helps us get restorative sleep without those horrible awakenings during the night. This idea is backed up by a review of factors associated with variation in sleep–wake patterns.[43] It was found that people who had greater variation had poorer sleep and more symptoms of insomnia. They also had greater symptoms of stress and depression. We should ideally keep things the same at the weekends too, to avoid social jetlag. While keeping bedtime consistent is good as a rule, the odd lie-in can also help us recover from a stressful week during which we have not had ample opportunity to sleep well. After all, we don't want to get into sleep debt.

If we do, it's best to try to pay it back rather than let it accumulate. This is not straightforward, however, as if the debt is large we don't seem to have the option to repay it all. This was demonstrated in the classic study of Randy Gardner, discussed in Chapter 1, who was sleep deprived for 264 hours in the name of science.[44] If his nightly sleep requirement was an average nine hours a night for a 17-year-old, he had around 99 hours of missed sleep to catch up on (nine hours of missed sleep for 11 days)! Yet, when he was allowed to sleep, he did not fall into a 99 hour-long slumber, but started with a relatively paltry 15 hours of kip on the first night. By the third night this had dropped to just over nine hours. A week after the experiment he slept for just seven hours.[45] While he initially appeared to be catching up on some of the sleep he had missed, this process was a slow one. When researchers looked at the type of sleep he was getting, it seemed that his body was prioritising REM and deep NREM sleep over lighter sleep – perhaps reflecting the particular importance of these types of sleep. Overall, when we think about the need for consistency in our sleep–wake schedule, this needs to be balanced with that of getting enough kip.*

---

* It is sometimes recommend that we should try to avoid more than two hours' difference in wake time between days that we are working and days that we are not. A consistent wake time is important to promote undisturbed and restorative sleep.

Abandon your inner hipster and get an early night

For some, parties, nightclubs and associated opportunities for amusement on the night bus are replaced with an early night as we age. But is this a reason to lament the end of our misspent youth, or should we be embracing these newfound early nights? Certainly, there is evidence that the time we go to bed is linked to the amount of sleep that we get. In a study mentioned in Chapter 7, a smartphone app was used to obtain information about sleep from adults around the world.[46] People in different countries slept for different lengths of time – with those from the UK sleeping for longer periods than those from Brazil, for example. When exploring the data a little further, it became very clear that key to driving the length of sleep that someone gets was bedtime and not waking time. This has also been found in other age groups and, as discussed in Chapter 4, the amount of sleep an adolescent gets appears to be related to the bedtime set by parents.[47] The importance of bedtime for sleep length makes sense, as while we often have control over the time we turn in for the night, commitments during the day can mean that the time we wake up is non-negotiable. So an early bedtime might result in more sleep, which for most of us is not a bad thing.*

Get some rays in the days and avoid light at night

Light is the very best cue from our environment to help the clock strike in time with the world around us. Would one solution therefore be to follow the mavericks, up sticks and live in a tent in the middle of nowhere? Anne-Marie, a friend of mine, did just that. Sick of the rat race, she decided to live in a yurt in the UK countryside with her young son, where

---

* Bringing bedtime forward gradually might be a good idea for those who are not getting enough sleep. However, we should only go to bed earlier if we are able to sleep during that time. This would not be a useful tip for someone experiencing insomnia, as they might end up spending more time lying in bed awake.

she had no electricity, running water or heating. She lived naturally, in tune with day and night and the seasons, and reported sleeping better than ever before. Her experience of good sleep was corroborated by researchers from the USA, who conducted a series of experiments aimed at trying to understand more about the effect of light and dark on our sleep patterns and body clocks.[48] In one experiment, they assessed the sleep patterns of a group of people for a week. They then asked them to go camping in the Rocky Mountains in Colorado during the winter. The participants got their light only from the sun, moon and campfires. It was found that the campers went to bed around two and a half hours earlier, compared with when they had access to artificial light and other mod cons. Additionally, the campers slept for more than two hours longer each night compared with beforehand, and were more active in the daytime. Light is likely to explain some of these findings, and when camping the participants were exposed to 13 times more light than when at home. The dark nights probably helped too. The importance of light on our sleep provides a reminder of the value of getting out during the day as well as considering blackout blinds, eye masks and light dimmers at night. Even a small amount of light can influence our sleep, so if we decide to use electric alarm clocks, we should point them away from us as we sleep.

Cool down or warm up?

Before bed, some people like to get snuggly. I typically spend time in the evening lying on my sofa in my beloved ancient bathrobe, under a brown fleecy blanket. Others share this passion for bedtime heat too and might enjoy a steamy bath or embracing a hot water bottle to keep them toasty at night.

Despite this popular craving for bedtime heat, the advice here seems somewhat confusing. To get a good night's sleep we are advised to sleep in a cool environment. For people who like practical advice, a typical recommendation is that we set the temperature in our house to an arctic 16–19°C (around 60–67°F) for the ideal sleeping temperature in adults. Recommendations fluctuate somewhat and there are individual differences in terms of what different people find most comfortable. How we should set our thermostat also depends somewhat on whether we choose to sleep in a thick onesie or in the nude, on the tog of our duvet and our size. According to one simulation, it was estimated that your 'average man' (in terms of body mass, skin surface area and metabolism) might be comfortable setting his thermostat at just 15°C (59°F) while sleeping[49] – likely saving energy, and as a consequence money and the environment too. Keeping a cool environment while we sleep is most important at the very earliest stages of life, where becoming overheated has been proposed as a possible risk for sudden infant death syndrome.[50]

So how might we reconcile the advice that both a hot bath and a cool environment might lead to a good night's sleep? Perhaps the easiest way to explain this is to consider that the overall aim might be to lose heat from the centre of the body. Our temperature changes throughout the day. As the evening draws to a close our core body temperature dips, which coincides with the time we fall asleep.[51] Keeping our core cool makes sense, as disrupting our core body temperature has the potential to disrupt our sleep.

When the environment is cool our bodies are able to lose heat, so setting the thermostat low makes sense. But what about the hot bath? Attending survival skills courses we are told not to rub someone with hypothermia, or to put them in a hot bath. This is because when we rub the skin or warm it in a bath the blood vessels dilate. This means that more blood moves towards the skin and away from the centre of the body. This is dangerous if it happens too quickly, as might be the case for someone with hypothermia. When blood is near the skin it is more likely to lose heat. This process can therefore result in a reduction in our core body temperature, which is associated with falling asleep. But what about my ancient bathrobe? Should that be ditched? Regardless of the science, and for the sake of my marriage, the answer is emphatically yes.

Although temperature is important for sleep, it is given far less attention than light. In contrast to shutting blinds and dimming lights before bedtime, many of us won't have ever considered the thermostat setting before going to bed. But perhaps we are missing a trick. These issues need to be considered beyond the home, and it remains important for those designing and running hotels, hostels, hospitals, halls of residence, affordable housing and care homes, to think carefully about the light and temperature of the accommodation they are offering. This is not just for the comfort of their residents, but for the sake of their sleep.

Given the advantages of a cool environment for a happy trip to dreamland, perhaps we should be concerned about the effects of global warming on our sleep. In a study led by a scientist from Harvard, self-reported information about insufficient sleep in 750,000 participants was analysed alongside data on night-time temperatures.[52] There was an association between greater temperature at night and poorer sleep. The authors predict that with a projected increase in global temperature this could lead to elevated sleeplessness. Perhaps achieving blissful sleep is just another reason to do what we can to protect our beautiful planet.

Banish electronics

One implication of needing to keep cool when we sleep is that we might want to banish the electric blanket from our bedroom. However, the array of electronics to be banned goes much further than that. Letting your child have a television in their room might buy you adoration, but watching it late at night and falling asleep while it is on will do little for their sleep quality. Designing a television into the cupboard at the end of the bed might seem luxurious, but it has risks. In fact, watching TV shows can cause problems and the CEO of Netflix is reported to have claimed that sleep is its biggest competitor. This led the American Academy of Sleep Medicine to issue a statement encouraging users of streaming services to binge-watch responsibly. For example, they might want to filter blue light from tablets and phones, not watch devices in bed and turn off screens at least half an hour before they turn in for the night.[53]

Phones, tablets and perhaps even music systems should be taken out of the bedroom – allowing it to become an oasis of calm. Not only does the light emitted from tablets have the potential to create havoc for our sleep, but the arousal associated with a late-night call or an interesting app can cause problems too. In addition to avoiding electronics, ban the clock – as 'clock watching' when you can't sleep is guaranteed to keep you up. If you must have a clock in the bedroom, turn down its illumination if it's electronic.

Stay fresh

Some people love nothing more than fresh bed linen, and that is no bad thing. Think about the amount of time we spend in bed and the things that we do in this 30-odd square feet of space! It doesn't take long to turn a spring-fresh bed into a stink-pit. There are sweaty nights, fungal toenails, midnight feasts and hacking coughs. We shed millions of cells every day and they, together with bed mites, can build up over a short period, leaving a distinct sweatiness to the linen. In fact, the research examining the air pollutants we are exposed to while asleep makes for grim reading, and bacteria, fungi, allergens and pollutants from our mattresses can all share our sleep environment.[54] All of these things are unlikely to be conducive to optimal sleep and some people even see fresh sheets as synonymous with a good night's sleep. Indeed, in a bedroom poll by the National Sleep Foundation, 1,500 adults aged 25–55 were asked about their bedroom environment and their sleep.[55] More than 7 out of 10 people questioned reported getting a more comfortable night's sleep when they had 'sheets with a fresh scent'. Change your sheets regularly, or throw back the duvet in the morning and allow air to get to the bed, so any moisture generated during the night can dry out. Sleep might thank you.

Further considering air quality in the bedroom, it's noteworthy that many of us shut our windows and bedroom doors when we sleep. This is sometimes for practical reasons such as to protect us from the pollution, the noise of traffic or perhaps cockerels that could disturb our slumber. However, where possible, ventilating the bedroom has a number of advantages. It can let out condensation and reduce the chances of visible mould and mould spores developing, and with them associated risks for respiratory problems, allergies and asthma;[56] visible mould around the house has been associated with poorer sleep.[57] Opening the windows can also reduce the levels of carbon dioxide building up in our bedrooms and, via a small study, decreasing this has been linked with both improved sleep quality and daytime functioning.[58]

Deal with your family

Sleep and family often don't mix well. A snoring or duvet-hogging partner, or a trespassing child, is unlikely to do our sleep any favours and we must always consider sleep in the family context. We should be proactive in our choices. If a noisy partner is leading us to exhaustion and underperformance at work, could we park our head down elsewhere? If trespassing children make us grumpy, we could put them back in their beds each time they visit so this behaviour is not reinforced.

Animals are often considered part of the family and can sometimes have equal status to that of our children in their ability to test our sleep. A new puppy can give a new baby a run for its money when it comes to messing with a caregiver's slumber! Even older pets can disturb sleep and dogs can need a tinkle or a cuddle, or might literally run us through their dreams (REM paralysis seems to work less well in dogs compared with humans). A large proportion of us have pets and around half of those that do let them sleep in the bedroom.[59] Whereas this can play havoc with our sleep, certain benefits have also been claimed. In line with the idea that we need to feel safe to sleep it's been argued that having a dog or cat can allow us to feel guarded and thus sleep soundly. A study conducted by researchers from the USA examined the effects of dogs on our sleep.[60] Forty adults and their dogs wore sleep trackers for seven nights. Having a dog in the bedroom was associated with 81 per cent sleep efficiency,* meaning that on average owners spent this proportion of their time in bed actually sleeping.† When the researchers examined this in more detail, they found that having dogs in the bedroom, but not the bed, was associated with slightly, but significantly greater sleep efficiency (83 per cent) than when dogs slept in the bed (80 per cent). One conclusion might be that if we do decide to keep Hazel the bulldog in our bedroom, it might be a good idea to make sure that her sweet spot is on the floor.

Don't let sleep become 'a thing'

We know that problems with our sleep, whether it is too short or long, disrupted or disordered, are often linked to other problems. However, we also need to let it go, as the way we think about our sleep is important in whether it ends up becoming a chronic issue.[62] If we don't sleep well one night, that doesn't necessarily mean that there is an escalating problem. After all, how many people can say they have *never* experienced a night of poor sleep? Mental or physical illness, or a bad day at the office, is not just down to poor sleep. Multiple factors are likely to have contributed. We should try to be relaxed about our sleep, as ideally it should be a pleasure, not a source of stress. Some issues affecting sleep, such as age, are outside our

---

* To calculate your own sleep efficiency you need to add up the total time you actually sleep, divided by the time you spend in bed. If you spend eight hours asleep but 10 hours in bed, your efficiency would be 80 per cent.
† To help further contextualise these findings, the National Sleep Foundation considers 85 per cent to represent good sleep quality in adults. It has been proposed that a sleep efficiency of 74 per cent or less does not signify good sleep quality in most age groups (except for young adults).[61]

control. Perhaps after following good sleep practices – and seeking help for any difficulties that we have – we should try acceptance. Ironically, it might be that if people are more accepting of sleeping poorly, this might prevent them from engaging in behaviours that could be inadvertently fuelling the problem and even result in improved sleep quality.[63]

Have sweet dreams

For some, getting a wonderful night's sleep may require more than sleeping soundly for an adequate period of time. A perfect kip may also include fantastical dreams that we simply don't want to end. We might want to fly high or swoop low with the flick of a limb. Some people wish they had more control over their dreams, to make them last longer or progress in a different way. Lucid dreaming involves just that – and over half of the population are lucky enough to have experienced one in their lifetime, with around a quarter reporting one or more a month.[64] Allan Hobson, an emeritus professor of psychiatry at Harvard Medical School, discussed in Chapter 1, and one of the biggest names in the field of dreaming research, described a period in the 1960s where he could use lucid dreams to sleep with whomever he pleased.[65] When you look at the brain activity of those experiencing lucid dreams you can see it is a state that involves components of both being awake and dreaming, hence creating this unusual in-between condition.

What techniques are useful for those who are keen to have a lucid dream? Lots of different methods have been developed, including cognitive approaches such as 'reality checks'.[66] This involves asking ourselves during the day whether we are dreaming or awake. This can help to create awareness of our state during sleep so that we can then actively take control of our dreams.

Other techniques include using stimulation, such as light, sound or water during REM sleep. For example, we could play the words 'this is a dream' while we are dreaming. The aim here is for the dreamer to obtain some awareness of being asleep and then to control the dream.[66] Snoozing after the alarm goes off provides another technique that could help us achieve a lucid dream,[67] with the possibility that some of our waking brain activity is carried back into our dream. The bad news for anyone keen to enjoy a lucid dream is that there has not been a great deal of support for these different techniques,[66] so these dreams might not be straightforward to achieve. For those lucky enough to enjoy the ability of dreaming lucidly – use it wisely.

The pill

The aim of this book is to share information about an incredible third of our lives – the time we spend asleep. If people obtain superior sleep, or enjoy it more after reading about it, even better! Perhaps we should take a moment to reflect on whether there is more we can do to prioritise our sleep and that of loved ones. We may decide to go to bed rather than watch an extra episode of that box set, or maybe we'll make that long-overdue investment in a blackout blind or banish pesky electronics from the bedroom.

But what if there was a different option? What if there were a pill or injection that could remove our need for sleep? This is currently unrealistic – but only a few decades back so was the internet as we know it today. Furthermore, there are already drugs that allow us to stay awake for long periods and avoid sleep. One example is modafinil – a drug sometimes prescribed for those with narcolepsy, to help patients stay awake and alert.[68] This has also been used to treat daytime sleepiness in others, such as shift workers or those suffering from sleep apnoea, or restless legs syndrome. It is sometimes referred to as the 'smart pill', as it can provide neuroenhancement – bolstering certain brain processes in healthy individuals[69] – although it is not without risks. It has been mooted over some time that we're not far away from developing drugs that would drastically reduce our need for sleep.[70]

What if we really could obliterate the need for sleep altogether? This thought experiment is not new,[71] and is described by the eminent sleep scientist Professor Jim Horne in his excellent book *Sleepfaring*. Here I outline and slightly extend Horne's idea. This pill could be a wonderful thing. We would not have exhausted children causing havoc in restaurants or on long flights, and bedtime struggles would be a thing of the past. We would never experience another nightmare. Huan would no longer need to worry about her daughter Lin sleepwalking out of hotel rooms at night (Chapter 3). Mrs Sinclair would not wake up paralysed and fearful (Chapter 3). We wouldn't worry that our heads might explode during the night. My husband would rejoice in never again having to see me plod the house in that ancient bathrobe.

We would have time, glorious time. A 90-year-old would have enjoyed an extra 30 years of life spent awake. Perhaps parents would have time to play with their children before school instead of barking instructions to get everyone to their destinations on time. Our bosses would be pleased with the increased time we could dedicate to our jobs. Conversations between partners would have time to flourish!

However, perhaps there is something pleasing about tired children. Without sleep, the joys of reading children bedtime stories would be gone. And as the witticism goes, 'Parents love their children most of all when they are fast asleep.' Would these ever-so-wide-awake children be loved that little bit less? The heavenly gap between children's bedtime and that of their parents would be lost. Would there ever be a time that adults could tidy faster than young children could create a mess? Being tired in the morning allows some of us to indulge in our first exquisite coffee of the day. At night it encourages consumption of a glass of wine because we know our brains aren't going to achieve much anyway. Tiredness gives us a valuable justification for relaxing with a book or in front of the TV. Going to bed is a reason to change our clothes. Some people love nothing more than getting into fresh pyjamas and sinking under fresh linen. There can be something confirmatory about lying next to a partner at night, even when we are too tired to interact. There is exultation when waking from a nightmare and appreciating what is not. A shared day and night encourages coordination of people within a society, dancing through their lives in harmony. England on a sunny day is a wonderful place. There is unity and joy that the clouds and rain have gone. But a world with constant sunshine would provide a drought, so what would a world without sleep look like?

And, would this pill really allow us to see our partners more? Businesses might expect more from their staff. Would Rakesh ever be allowed to return home to his sleepless wife (Chapter 7)? Why bother allowing employees time to go home to sleep when they no longer need it? Instead, businesses could strongly encourage that staff waive their right to sleep and stay at work all the time. And, even if alertness was maintained, just how good would we be at our jobs without time away to reflect and 'sleep on it'? Would we ever take stock of the day? New discoveries attributable to sleep or dreaming would never evolve. My friend Michelle, who believes that she can predict what will happen in life via her dreams, would be left with her third eye spinning (Chapter 3).

And what about our dreams? When flesh is gone, dreams offer us a final chance of being reunited with loved ones. So, my question is this: what if we could create a pill that could obliterate permanently the need to sleep? A safe pill that would allow us to restore our bodies, remove toxins from our brains, learn, remember and forget, and to feel rejuvenated, ready to cope with the emotional assaults of the day. We could bid a final farewell to sleep, that friend who is sometimes controversial but has always been by our side. Thinking back to sleep throughout our life, I wonder if the many people with whom I discussed sleep at different stages of life would take this pill? Would Mitch, the father of young Charlie diagnosed with global developmental delay, benefit from this? How about Roger, who struggles so greatly with his insomnia, or Guy the shift worker? And what about the elderly couple Marco and Maria who over the years have come to fall out of love with bedtime? If the pill were on my pillow tonight, I know what I would do. What about you?

References

Prologue

1 Harvey, A. G., Gregory, A. M. & Bird, C. 2002. The role of cognitive processes in sleep disturbance: a comparison of Japanese and English university students. *Behavioural and Cognitive Psychotherapy* 30:259–70.

2 Gregory, A. M., Caspi, A., Eley, T. C., et al. 2005. Prospective longitudinal associations between persistent sleep problems in childhood and anxiety and depression disorders in adulthood. *Journal of Abnormal Child Psychology* 33:157–63.

3 Gregory, A. M., Rijsdijk, F. V., Dahl, R. E., et al. 2006. Associations between sleep problems, anxiety and depression in twins at 8 years of age. *Pediatrics* 118:1124–32.

4 Gregory, A. M., Willis, T. A., Wiggs, L., et al. 2008. Presleep arousal and sleep disturbances in children. *Sleep* 31:1745–7.

5 Barclay, N. L., Eley, T. C., Buysse, D. J., et al. 2010. Diurnal preference and sleep quality: same genes? A study of young adult twins. *Chronobiology International* 27:278–96.

6 McMakin, D. L., Dahl, R. E., Buysse, D. J., et al. 2016. The impact of experimental sleep restriction on affective functioning in social and nonsocial contexts among adolescents. *Journal of Child Psychology and Psychiatry* 57:1027–37.

7 Denis D., French, C. C., Rowe, R., et al. 2015. A twin and molecular genetics study of sleep paralysis and associated factors. *Journal of Sleep Research* 24:438–46.

8 Troxel, W. M., Robles, T. F., Hall, M., et al. 2007. Marital quality and the marital bed: examining the covariation between relationship quality and sleep. *Sleep Medicine Reviews* 11:389–404.

Chapter 1: Sleep 101

1 Gent, T. & Adamantidis, A. 2017. Anaesthesia and sleep: Where are we now? *Clinical and Translational Neuroscience* https://doi.org/10.1177/2514183X17726281.

2 Borbely, A. A. 1982. A two process model of sleep regulation. *Human Neurobiology* 1:195–204.

3 Allada, R., Cirelli, C. & Sehgal, A. 2017. Molecular mechanisms of sleep homeostasis in flies and mammals. *Cold Spring Harbor Perspectives in Biology* 9:a027730.

4 Clark, I. & Landolt, H. P. 2017. Coffee, caffeine, and sleep: a systematic review of epidemiological studies and randomized controlled trials. *Sleep Medicine Reviews* 31:70–8.

5 Takahashi, J. S. 2017. Transcriptional architecture of the mammalian circadian clock. *Nature Reviews Genetics* 18:164–79.

6 Rechtschaffen, A. & Bergmann, B. M. 2002. Sleep deprivation in the rat: an update of the 1989 paper. *Sleep* 25:18–24.

7 Llorens, F., Zarranz, J. J., Fischer, A., et al. 2017. Fatal familial insomnia: clinical aspects and molecular alterations. *Current Neurology and Neuroscience Reports* 17:30.

8 Ross, J. J. 1965. Neurological findings after prolonged sleep deprivation. *Archives of Neurology* 12:399–403.

9 Lockley, S. W. & Foster, R. G. 2012. *Sleep: A Very Short Introduction.* Oxford University Press, Oxford.

10 Carey, H. V., Andrews, M. T. & Martin, S. L. 2003. Mammalian hibernation: cellular and molecular responses to depressed metabolism and low temperature. *Physiological Reviews* 83:1153–81.

11 Jung, C. M., Melanson, E. L., Frydendall, E. J., et al. 2011. Energy expenditure during sleep, sleep deprivation and sleep following sleep deprivation in adult humans. *Journal of Physiology* 589:235–44.

12 Mascetti, G. G. 2016. Unihemispheric sleep and asymmetrical sleep: behavioral, neurophysiological, and functional perspectives. *Nature and Science of Sleep* 8:221–37.

13 Schmidt, M. H. 2014. The energy allocation function of sleep: a unifying theory of sleep, torpor, and continuous wakefulness. *Neuroscience and Biobehavioral Reviews* 47:122–53.

14 Xie, L., Kang, H., Xu, Q., et al. 2013. Sleep drives metabolite clearance from the adult brain. *Science* 342:373–7.

15 Vorster, A. P. & Born, J. 2015. Sleep and memory in mammals, birds and invertebrates. *Neuroscience and Biobehavioral Reviews* 50:103–19.

16 Wagner, U., Gais, S., Haider, H., et al. 2004. Sleep inspires insight. *Nature* 427:352–5.

17 Tononi, G. & Cirelli, C. 2014. Sleep and the price of plasticity: from synaptic and cellular homeostasis to memory consolidation and integration. *Neuron* 81:12–34.

18 Walker, M. P. & van der Helm, E. 2009. Overnight therapy? The role of sleep in emotional brain processing. *Psychological Bulletin* 135:731–48.

19 Barras, C. 2016. What is the real reason we sleep? www.bbc. com/earth/story/20160317-what-is-the-real-reason-we-sleep.

20 Goldstein, A. N. & Walker, M. P. 2014. The role of sleep in emotional brain function. *Annual Review of Clinical Psychology* 10:679–708.

21 Kurth, S., Ringli, M., Geiger, A., et al. 2010. Mapping of cortical activity in the first two decades of life: a high-density sleep electroencephalogram study. *Journal of Neuroscience* 30:13211–9.

22 Mander, B.A., Rao, V., Lu, B., et al. 2013. Prefrontal atrophy, disrupted NREM slow waves and impaired hippocampal-dependent memory in aging. *Nature Neuroscience* 16:357–64.

23 Siegel, J. M. 2009. Sleep – Opinion: sleep viewed as a state of adaptive inactivity. *Nature Reviews Neuroscience* 10:747–53.

24 Dahl, R. 1982. *The BFG*. Jonathan Cape, London.

25 Cartwright, R. 2008. The contribution of the psychology of sleep and dreaming to understand sleep-disordered patients. *Sleep Medicine Clinics* 3:157–66.

26 Hobson, J. A. & McCarley, R. W. 1977. The brain as a dream state generator – an activation–synthesis hypothesis of dream process. *American Journal of Psychiatry* 134:1335–48.

27 Hobson, J. A. 2009. REM sleep and dreaming: towards a theory of protoconsciousness. *Nature Reviews Neuroscience* 10: 803–813.

Chapter 2: Sleeping Like a Baby: Sleep in the First Years of Life

1 Paruthi S., Brooks L. J., D'Ambrosio, C., et al. 2016. Recommended amount of sleep for pediatric populations: a consensus statement of the American academy of sleep medicine. *Journal of Clinical Sleep Medicine* 12:785–6.

2   Fifer, W. P., Byrd, D. L., Kaku, M., et al. 2010. Newborn
    infants learn during sleep. *Proceedings of the National
    Academy of Sciences of the United States of America*
    107:10320–3.
3   Mindell, J. A., Sadeh, A., Wiegand, B., et al. 2010. Cross-
    cultural differences in infant and toddler sleep. *Sleep Medicine*
    11:274–80.
4   Lee, K. A. & Rosen, L. A. 2012. Sleep and human
    development. Edited by Morin, C. M. & Espie, C. A. 2012.
    The Oxford Handbook of Sleep and Sleep Disorders. Oxford
    University Press, Oxford.
5   Mirmiran, M., Maas, Y. G. H. & Ariagno, R. L. 2003.
    Development of fetal and neonatal sleep and circadian
    rhythms. *Sleep Medicine Reviews* 7:321–34.
6   Engler, A. C., Hadash, A., Shehadeh, N., et al. 2012.
    Breastfeeding may improve nocturnal sleep and reduce
    infantile colic: potential role of breast milk melatonin.
    European Journal of Pediatrics 171:729–32.
7   Ferber, R. 2013. *Solve Your Child's Sleep Problems*. Vermilion,
    London.
8   Marks, G. A., Shaffery, J. P., Oksenberg, A., et al. 1995.
    A functional role for REM-sleep in brain maturation.
    Behavioural Brain Research 69:1–11.
9   Dumoulin Bridi, M. C. D., Aton, S. J., Seibt, J., et al. 2015.
    Rapid eye movement sleep promotes cortical plasticity in the
    developing brain. *Science Advances* 1:e1500105.
10 Carnegie, D. 2006. *How to Win Friends and Influence People*.
    Vermilion, London.
11 Plomin, R., DeFries, J. C., Knopik, V. S., et al. 2013.
    Behavioral Genetics. 6th ed. Worth Publishers, New York.
12 Fisher, A., van Jaarsveld, C. H. M., Llewellyn, C. H., et al.
    2012. Genetic and environmental influences on infant sleep.
    Pediatrics 129:1091–6.
13 Barclay, N. L. & Gregory, A. M. 2013. Quantitative genetic
    research on sleep: a review of normal sleep, sleep
    disturbances and associated emotional, behavioural, and
    health-related difficulties. *Sleep Medicine Reviews* 17:29–40.
14 Marinelli, M., Pappa, I., Bustamante, M., et al. 2016.
    Heritability and genome-wide association analyses of sleep
    duration in children: the EAGLE consortium. *Sleep*
    39:1859–69.

15 Hammerschlag, A. R., Stringer, S., de Leeuw, C. A., et al. 2017. Genome-wide association analysis of insomnia complaints identifies risk genes and genetic overlap with psychiatric and metabolic traits. *Nature Genetics* 49:1584–92.

16 Mindell, J. A., Li, A. M., Sadeh, A., et al. 2015. Bedtime routines for young children: a dose-dependent association with sleep outcomes. *Sleep* 38:717–22.

17 O'Connor, T. G., Caprariello, P., Blackmore, E. R., et al. 2007. Prenatal mood disturbance predicts sleep problems in infancy and toddlerhood. *Early Human Development* 83:451–8.

18 Wiggs, L. 2007. Are children getting enough sleep? Implications for parents. *Sociological Research Online* 12:13.

19 Friedman, U. 2015. How to snore in Korean: the mystery of onomatopocia around the world. www.theatlantic.com/international/archive/2015/11/onomatopoeia-world-languages/415824.

20 Hirshkowitz, M., Whiton, K., Albert, S. M., et al. 2015. National Sleep Foundation's sleep time duration recommendations: methodology and results summary. *Sleep Health* 1:40–3.

21 Midgley, F. 2016. Cot death: how Anne Diamond helped save thousands of babies. www.bbc.co.uk/news/uk-england-berkshire-37908627.

22 Lullaby Trust. 2017. www.lullabytrust.org.uk/wp-content/uploads/Facts-and-Figures-for-2015-released-2017.pdf.

23 Moon, R. Y., Darnall, R. A., Feldman-Winter, L., et al. 2016. SIDS and other sleep-related infant deaths: evidence base for 2016 updated recommendations for a safe infant sleeping environment. *Pediatrics* 138:e20162940.

24 Kreth, M., Shikany, T., Lenker, C., et al. 2017. Safe sleep guideline adherence in nationwide marketing of infant cribs and products. *Pediatrics* 139:e20161729.

25 Noack, R. 2015. Why babies should sleep in cardboard boxes, explained in 2 charts. www.washingtonpost.com/news/worldviews/wp/2015/11/10/why-babies-should-sleep-in-cardboard-boxes-explained-in-2-charts/?utm_term=.bc3eadd66383.

26 BBC. 2017. Cot death charity raises doubts over baby boxes. www.bbc.co.uk/news/uk-40810110.

27 Mindell, J. A., Kuhn, B., Lewin, D. S., et al. 2006.
    Behavioral treatment of bedtime problems and night
    wakings in infants and young children – an American
    Academy of Sleep Medicine review. *Sleep* 29:1263–76.
28 Williams, S. E. & Horst, J. S. 2014. Goodnight book: sleep
    consolidation improves word learning via story books.
    Frontiers in Psychology 5:184.
29 Meltzer, L. J. & Mindell, J. A. 2014. Systematic review and
    meta-analysis of behavioral interventions for pediatric
    insomnia. *Journal of Pediatric Psychology* 39:932–48.
30 Hiscock, H., Bayer, J. K., Hampton, A., et al. 2008. Long-
    term mother and child mental health effects of a population-
    based infant sleep intervention: cluster-randomized,
    controlled trial. *Pediatrics* 122:e621–e627.
31 Hiscock, H. & Fisher, J. 2015. Sleeping like a baby? Infant
    sleep: impact on caregivers and current controversies. *Journal
    of Paediatrics and Child Health* 51:361–4.
32 Gradisar, M., Jackson, K., Spurrier, N. J., et al. 2016.
    Behavioral interventions for infant sleep problems: a
    randomized controlled trial. *Pediatrics* 137:e20151486.
33 Price, A. M. H., Wake, M., Ukoumunne, O. C., et al. 2012.
    Five-year follow-up of harms and benefits of behavioral infant
    sleep intervention: randomized trial. *Pediatrics* 130:643–51.
34 Middlemiss, W., Granger, D. A., Goldberg, W. A., et al.
    2012. Asynchrony of mother–infant hypothalamic–
    pituitary–adrenal axis activity following extinction of infant
    crying responses induced during the transition to sleep. *Early
    Human Development* 88:227–32.
35 Price, A., Hiscock, H. & Gradisar, M. 2013. Let's help parents help
    themselves: a letter to the editor supporting the safety of
    behavioural sleep techniques. *Early Human Development* 89:39–40.
36 Middlemiss, W., Granger, D. A. & Goldberg, W. A. 2013.
    Response to 'Let's help parents help themselves: a letter to
    the editor supporting the safety of behavioural sleep
    techniques'. *Early Human Development* 89:41–2.

Chapter 3: Preschool and School-Aged Children: The Rainbow of Sleep Problems

1 Paruthi. S, Brooks L. J., D'Ambrosio, C., et al. 2016.
    Recommended amount of sleep for pediatric populations: a

consensus statement of the American Academy of Sleep Medicine. *Journal of Clinical Sleep Medicine* 12:785–6.

2 American Academy of Sleep Medicine. 2014. *International Classification of Sleep Disorders.* 3rd ed. American Academy of Sleep Medicine, Darien, Illinois.

3 Mansbach, A. 2011. *Go the Fuck to Sleep.* Akashic, New York.

4 Van Geel, M., Goemans, A. & Vedder, P. H. 2016. The relation between peer victimization and sleeping problems: a meta-analysis. *Sleep Medicine Reviews* 27:89–95.

5 Sadeh, A. 1996. Stress, trauma, and sleep in children. *Child and Adolescent Psychiatric Clinics of North America* 5:685–700.

6 Kajeepeta, S., Gelaye, B., Jackson, C. L., et al. 2015. Adverse childhood experiences are associated with adult sleep disorders: a systematic review. *Sleep Medicine* 16:320–30.

7 Harvey, A. G. 2002. A cognitive model of insomnia. *Behaviour Research & Therapy* 40:869–93.

8 Gregory, A. M., Cox, J., Crawford, M. R., et al. 2009. Dysfunctional beliefs and attitudes about sleep in children. *Journal of Sleep Research* 18:422–6.

9 Gregory, A. M., Noone, D. M., Eley, T. C., et al. 2010. Catastrophising and symptoms of sleep disturbances in children. *Journal of Sleep Research* 19:175–82.

10 Gregory, A. M., Willis, T. A., Wiggs, L., et al. 2008. Pre-sleep arousal and sleep disturbances in children. *Sleep* 31:1745–7.

11 Ehrlin, C-J. F. 2015. *The Rabbit Who Wants to Fall Asleep.* Ladybird, London.

12 Alfano, C. A., Pina, A. A., Zerr, A. A., et al. 2010. Pre-sleep arousal and sleep problems of anxiety-disordered youth. *Child Psychiatry and Human Development* 41:156–67.

13 De Houwer, J., Teige-Mocigemba, S., Spruyt, A., et al. 2009. Implicit measures: a normative analysis and review. *Psychological Bulletin* 135:347–68.

14 Schlarb, A. A., Bihlmaier, I., Velten-Schurian, K., et al. 2016. Short- and long-term effects of CBT-I in groups for school-age children suffering from chronic insomnia: the KiSS-program. *Behavioral Sleep Medicine.* www.tandfonline. com/doi/abs/10.1080/15402002.2016.1228642.

15 Brockmann, P. E., Diaz, B., Damiani, F., et al. 2016. Impact of television on the quality of sleep in preschool children. *Sleep Medicine* 20:140-4.

16 Blunden, S. L., Chapman, J. & Rigney, G. A. 2012. Are sleep education programs successful? The case for improved and consistent research efforts. *Sleep Medicine Reviews* 16:355–70.

17 Curti, M. 1966. The American exploration of dreams and dreamers. *Journal of the History of Ideas* 27:391–416.

18 Sandor, P., Szakadat, S. & Bodizs, R. 2016. The development of cognitive and emotional processing as reflected in children's dreams: active self in an eventful dream signals better neuropsychological skills. *Dreaming* 26:58–78.

19 Floress, M. T., Kuhn, B. R., Bernas, R. S., et al. 2016. Nightmare prevalence, distress, and anxiety among young children. *Dreaming* 26:280–92.

20 Mindell, J. A. & Owens, J. A. 2015. *A Clinical Guide to Pediatric Sleep: Diagnosis and management of sleep problems.* 3rd ed. Wolters Kluwer, Philadelphia.

21 Hansen, K., Hoefling, V., Kroener-Borowik, T., et al. 2013. Efficacy of psychological interventions aiming to reduce chronic nightmares: a meta-analysis. *Clinical Psychology Review* 33:146–55.

22 De Cock, V. C. 2016. Sleepwalking. *Current Treatment Options in Neurology* 18:6.

23 Hoban, T. F. 2010. Sleep disorders in children. *Annals of the New York Academy of Sciences* 1184:1–14.

24 Silverman, R. 2013. Rachel Weisz and I ban technology from our bedroom, says Daniel Craig. www.telegraph.co.uk/culture/film/10297448/Rachel-Weisz-and-I-ban-technology-from-our-bedroom-says-Daniel-Craig.html.

25 Bonuck, K., Freeman, K., Chervin, R. D., et al. 2012. Sleep-disordered breathing in a population-based cohort: behavioral outcomes at 4 and 7 years. *Pediatrics* 129:e857–e865.

26 Guaita, M. & Hogl, B. 2016. Current treatments of bruxism. *Current Treatment Options in Neurology* 18:10.

27 Beckett, C., Bredenkamp, D., Castle, J., et al. 2002. Behavior patterns associated with institutional deprivation: a study of children adopted from Romania. *Journal of Developmental and Behavioral Pediatrics* 23:297–303.

28 Kuwertz-Broking, E. & von Gontard, A. 2017. Clinical management of nocturnal enuresis. *Pediatric Nephrology*, https://doi.org/10.1007/s00467-017-3778-1.

29 Sarici, H., Telli, O., Ozgur, B. C., et al. 2016. Prevalence of nocturnal enuresis and its influence on quality of life in school-aged children. *Journal of Pediatric Urology* 12:159. e1–159.e6.

30 Al-Zaben, F. N. & Sehlo, M. G. 2015. Punishment for bedwetting is associated with child depression and reduced quality of life. *Child Abuse & Neglect* 43:22–9.

31 Schlomer, B., Rodriguez, E., Weiss, D., et al. 2013. Parental beliefs about nocturnal enuresis causes, treatments, and the need to seek professional medical care. *Journal of Pediatric Urology* 9:1043–8.

32 Myint, M., Adam, A., Herath, S., et al. 2016. Mobile phone applications in management of enuresis: the good, the bad, and the unreliable! *Journal of Pediatric Urology* 12:112.e1–112.e6.

33 Longstreth, W. T., Koepsell, T. D., Ton, T. G., et al. 2007. The epidemiology of narcolepsy. *Sleep* 30:13–26.

34 Partinen, M., Saarenpaa-Heikkila, O., Ilveskoski, I., et al. 2012. Increased incidence and clinical picture of childhood narcolepsy following the 2009 H1N1 pandemic vaccination campaign in Finland. *PloS One* 7:e33723.

35 Denis, D., French, C. C., Rowe, R., et al. 2015. A twin and molecular genetics study of sleep paralysis and associated factors. *Journal of Sleep Research* 24:438–46.

36 Jimenez-Genchi, A., Vila-Rodriguez, V. M., Sanchez-Rojas, F., et al. 2009. Sleep paralysis in adolescents: the 'a dead body climbed on top of me' phenomenon in Mexico. *Psychiatry and Clinical Neurosciences* 63:546–9.

37 Sharpless, B. A. 2017. *Unusual and Rare Psychological Disorders: A handbook for clinical practice and research*. Oxford University Press, New York.

38 Sharpless, B. A. 2014. Exploding head syndrome. *Sleep Medicine Reviews* 18:489–93.

39 Meltzer, L. J. & McLaughlin, V. 2015. *Pediatric Sleep Problems: A clinician's guide to behavioral interventions*. American Psychological Association, Washington, DC.

40 Ferber, R. 2013. *Solve Your Child's Sleep Problems*. Vermilion, London.

41 Quine, L. 1997. *Solving Children's Sleep Problems: A step-by-step guide for parents*. Beckett Karlson Ltd, Huntingdon.

42 Huebner, D. 2008. *What to Do When You Dread Your Bed: A kid's guide to overcoming problems with sleep.* Magination Press, Washington, DC.

43 Bruni, O., Onso-Alconada, D., Besag, F., et al. 2015. Current role of melatonin in pediatric neurology: clinical recommendations. *European Journal of Paediatric Neurology* 19:122–33.

44 Waldron, A. Y., Spark, M. J. & Dennis, C. M. 2016. The use of melatonin by children: parents' perspectives. *Journal of Clinical Sleep Medicine* 12:1395–401.

45 Kennaway, D. J. 2015. Paediatric use of melatonin. *European Journal of Paediatric Neurology* 19:489–90.

46 Erland, L. A. E. & Saxena, P. K. 2017. Melatonin natural health products and supplements: presence of serotonin and significant variability of melatonin content. *Journal of Clinical Sleep Medicine* 13:275–81.

47 Byars, K. C., Yolton, K., Rausch, J., et al. 2012. Prevalence, patterns, and persistence of sleep problems in the first 3 years of life. *Pediatrics* 129:e276–e284.

48 Quach, J., Hiscock, H., Canterford, L., et al. 2009. Outcomes of child sleep problems over the school-transition period: Australian population longitudinal study. *Pediatrics* 123:1287–92.

Chapter 4: Laaazzzy? Adolescents' Sleep

1 Paruthi, S., Brooks, L. J., D'Ambrosio, C., et al. 2016. Recommended amount of sleep for pediatric populations: a consensus statement of the American Academy of Sleep Medicine. *Journal of Clinical Sleep Medicine* 12:785–6.

2 Crowley, S. J., Acebo, C. & Carskadon, M. A. 2007. Sleep, circadian rhythms, and delayed phase in adolescence. *Sleep Medicine* 8:602–12.

3 Dorofaeff, T. F. & Denny, S. 2006. Sleep and adolescence. Do New Zealand teenagers get enough? *Journal of Paediatrics and Child Health* 42:515–20.

4 Park, Y. M., Matsumoto, K., Seo, Y. J., et al. 2002. Changes of sleep or waking habits by age and sex in Japanese. *Perceptual and Motor Skills* 94:1199–213.

5   Saarenpaa-Heikkika, O. A., Rintahaka, P. J., Laippala, P. J.,
    et al. 1995. Sleep habits and disorders in Finnish
    schoolchildren. *Journal of Sleep Research* 4:173–82.
6   Hagenauer, M. H., Perryman, J. I., Lee, T. M., et al. 2009.
    Adolescent changes in the homeostatic and circadian
    regulation of sleep. *Developmental Neuroscience* 31:276–84.
7   Crowley, S. J., Cain, S. W., Burns, A. C., et al. 2015.
    Increased sensitivity of the circadian system to light in early/
    mid-puberty. *Journal of Clinical Endocrinology & Metabolism*
    100:4067–73.
8   Carskadon, M. A., Labyak, S. E., Acebo, C., et al. 1999.
    Intrinsic circadian period of adolescent humans measured in
    conditions of forced desynchrony. *Neuroscience Letters*
    260:129–32.
9   McGinnis, M. Y., Lumia, A. R., Tetel, M. J., et al. 2007.
    Effects of anabolic androgenic steroids on the development
    and expression of running wheel activity and circadian
    rhythms in male rats. *Physiology & Behavior* 92:1010–8.
10 Taylor, D. J., Jenni, O. G., Acebo, C., et al. 2005. Sleep
    tendency during extended wakefulness: insights into
    adolescent sleep regulation and behavior. *Journal of Sleep
    Research* 14:239–44.
11 Jenni, O. G., Achermann, P. & Carskadon, M. A. 2005.
    Homeostatic sleep regulation in adolescents. *Sleep*
    28:1446–54.
12 Carskadon, M. A. 2011. Sleep in adolescents: the perfect
    storm. *Pediatric Clinics of North America* 58:637–47.
13 Teenagers debunked. 2015. Teenagers debunked. https://
    thepsychologist.bps.org.uk/teenagers-debunked.
14 Samson, D. R., Crittenden, A. N., Mabulla, I. A., et al. 2017.
    Chronotype variation drives night-time sentinel-like
    behaviour in hunter-gatherers. *Proceedings of the Royal Society
    B-Biological Sciences* 284:20170967.
15 Ellis, B. J., Del Giudice, M., Dishion, T. J., et al. 2012. The
    evolutionary basis of risky adolescent behavior: implications
    for science, policy, and practice. *Developmental Psychology*
    48:598–623.
16 Owens, J. A., Dearth-Wesley, T., Lewin, D., et al. 2016. Self-
    regulation and sleep duration, sleepiness, and chronotype in
    adolescents. *Pediatrics* 138:e20161406.

17   Schlarb, A. A., Sopp, R., Ambiel, D., et al. 2014.
     Chronotype-related differences in childhood and adolescent
     aggression and antisocial behavior – A review of the
     literature. *Chronobiology International* 31:1–16.
18   Hasler, B. P., Franzen, P. L., de Zambotti, M., et al. 2017.
     Eveningness and later sleep timing are associated with
     greater risk for alcohol and marijuana use in adolescence:
     initial findings from the National Consortium on Alcohol
     and Neurodevelopment in Adolescence Study. *Alcoholism:
     Clinical and Experimental Research* 41:1154–65.
19   Muro, A., Freixanet, M. & Adan, A. 2012. Circadian
     typology and sensation seeking in adolescents. *Chronobiology
     International* 29:1376–82.
20   Barclay, N. L., Eley, T. C., Mill, J., et al. 2011. Sleep quality
     and diurnal preference in a sample of young adults:
     associations with 5HTTLPR, PER3, and CLOCK 3111.
     *American Journal of Medical Genetics Part B: Neuropsychiatric
     Genetics* 156:681–90.
21   Adan, A., Archer, S. N., Paz Hidalgo, M., et al. 2012.
     Circadian typology: a comprehensive review. *Chronobiology
     International* 29:1153–75.
22   Hu, Y., Shmygelska, A., Tran, D., et al. 2016. GWAS of
     89,283 individuals identifies genetic variants associated with
     self-reporting of being a morning person. *Nature
     Communications* 7:10448.
23   Jones, S. E., Tyrrell, J., Wood, A. R., et al. 2016. Genome-
     wide association analyses in 128,266 individuals identifies
     new morningness and sleep duration loci. *Plos Genetics*
     12:e1006125.
24   Burke, T. M., Markwald, R. R., Mchill, A. W., et al. 2015.
     Effects of caffeine on the human circadian clock in vivo and
     in vitro. *Science Translational Medicine* 7:305ra146.
25   Haynie, D. L., Lewin, D., Luk, J. W., et al. 2018. Beyond
     sleep duration: bidirectional associations between
     chronotype, social jetlag, and drinking behaviors in a
     longitudinal sample of US high school students. *Sleep.*
     zsx202, https://doi.org/10.1093/sleep/zsx202.
26   National Sleep Foundation. 2006. National Sleep Foundation
     Sleep in America poll. National Sleep Foundation,
     Washington, DC.

27 Buxton, O. M., Chang, A-M., Spilsbury, J. C., et al. 2015. Sleep in the modern family: protective family routines for child and adolescent sleep. *Sleep Health* 1:15–27.

28 Cain, N. & Gradisar, M. 2010. Electronic media use and sleep in school-aged children and adolescents: a review. *Sleep Medicine* 11:735–42.

29 Gradisar, M., Wolfson, A. R., Harvey, A. G., et al. 2013. The sleep and technology use of Americans: findings from the National Sleep Foundation's 2011 sleep in America poll. *Journal of Clinical Sleep Medicine* 9:1291–9.

30 LeGates, T. A., Fernandez, D. C. & Hattar, S. 2014. Light as a central modulator of circadian rhythms, sleep and affect. *Nature Reviews Neuroscience* 15:443–54.

31 Cheung, C. H. M., Bedford, R., De Urabain, I. R. S., et al. 2017. Daily touchscreen use in infants and toddlers is associated with reduced sleep and delayed sleep onset. *Scientific Reports* 7:46104.

32 Gringras, P., Middleton, B., Skene, D. J., et al. 2015. Bigger, brighter, bluer-better? Current light-emitting devices – adverse sleep properties and preventative strategies. *Frontiers in Public Health* 3:233.

33 Heath, M., Sutherland, C., Bartel, K., et al. 2014. Does one hour of bright or short-wavelength filtered tablet screenlight have a meaningful effect on adolescents' pre-bedtime alertness, sleep, and daytime functioning? *Chronobiology International* 31:496–505.

34 Wood, B., Rea, M. S., Plitnick, B., et al. 2013. Light level and duration of exposure determine the impact of self-luminous tablets on melatonin suppression. *Applied Ergonomics* 44:237–40.

35 Chang, A. M., Santhi, N., St Hilaire, M., et al. 2012. Human responses to bright light of different durations. *Journal of Physiology* 590:3103–12.

36 van der Lely, S., Frey, S., Garbazza, C., et al. 2015. Blue blocker glasses as a countermeasure for alerting effects of evening light-emitting diode screen exposure in male teenagers. *Journal of Adolescent Health* 56:113–9.

37 Gallagher, J. 2016. Praise for 'sleep-protecting' phones. www.bbc.co.uk/news/health-35311581.

38 Carlyle, R. 2012. Is your child really getting enough sleep? www.millpondsleepclinic.com/press-article/is-your-child-really-getting-enough-sleep.

39 Carter, B., Rees, P., Hale, L., et al. 2016. Association between portable screen-based media device access or use and sleep outcomes: a systematic review and meta-analysis. *Journal of the American Medical Association Pediatrics* 170:1202–8.

40 Mill, J. & Heijmans, B. T. 2013. From promises to practical strategies in epigenetic epidemiology. *Nature Reviews Genetics* 14:585–94.

41 Wong, C. C. Y., Parsons, M. J., Lester, K. J., et al. 2015. Epigenome-wide DNA methylation analysis of monozygotic twins discordant for diurnal preference. *Twin Research and Human Genetics* 18:662–9.

42 Taylor, A., Wright, H. R. & Lack, L. C. 2008. Sleeping-in on the weekend delays circadian phase and increases sleepiness the following week. *Sleep and Biological Rhythms* 6:172–9.

43 Harvey, A. G. 2016. A transdiagnostic intervention for youth sleep and circadian problems. *Cognitive and Behavioral Practice* 23:341–55.

44 Wittmann, M., Dinich, J., Merrow, M., et al. 2006. Social jetlag: misalignment of biological and social time. *Chronobiology International* 23:497–509.

45 Hasler, B. P., Dahl, R. E., Holm, S. M., et al. 2012. Weekend–weekday advances in sleep timing are associated with altered reward-related brain function in healthy adolescents. *Biological Psychology* 91:334–41.

46 Karatsoreos, I. N., Bhagat, S., Bloss, E. B., et al. 2011. Disruption of circadian clocks has ramifications for metabolism, brain, and behavior. *Proceedings of the National Academy of Sciences of the United States of America* 108:1657–62.

47 Parsons, M., Moffitt, T., Gregory, A., et al. 2015. Social jetlag, obesity and metabolic disorder: investigation in a cohort study. *International Journal of Obesity* 39:842–8.

48 Macrae, F. & Parry, L. 2015. Looking forward to your Saturday lie-in? Careful, it may be a health hazard: changes in sleep pattern between work days and weekend can raise chance of obesity and diabetes. www.dailymail.co.uk/health/article-2918139/Do-suffer-social-jetlag-two-hour-lie-weekend-increases-risk-OBESE-scientists-warn.

49 Broussard, J. L., Wroblewski, K., Kilkus, J. M., et al. 2016.
    Two nights of recovery sleep reverses the effects of short-term
    sleep restriction on diabetes risk. *Diabetes Care* 39:e40–e41.
50 Wahlstrom, K. 2010. School start time and sleepy teens.
    Archives of Pediatrics & Adolescent Medicine 164:676–7.
51 Wahlstrom, K. 2002. Changing times: findings from the first
    longitudinal study of later high school start times. *NASSP
    Bulletin* 86:3–21.
52 Danner, F. & Phillips, B. 2008. Adolescent sleep, school start
    times, and teen motor vehicle crashes. *Journal of Clinical Sleep
    Medicine* 4:533–5.
53 Minges, K. E. & Redeker, N. S. 2016. Delayed school start
    times and adolescent sleep: a systematic review of the
    experimental evidence. *Sleep Medicine Reviews* 28:86–95.
54 Hafner, M., Stepanck, M. & Troxel, W. M. 2017. *Later School
    Start Times in the U.S. An Economic analysis*. RAND,
    Cambridge.
55 Short, M. A., Gradisar, M., Wright, H., et al. 2011. Time for
    bed: parent-set bedtimes associated with improved sleep and
    daytime functioning in adolescents. *Sleep* 34:797–800.
56 Gangwisch, J. E., Babiss, L. A., Malaspina, D., et al. 2010.
    Earlier parental set bedtimes as a protective factor against
    depression and suicidal ideation. *Sleep* 33:97–106.
57 Dewald-Kaufmann, J. F., Oort, F. J. & Meijer, A. M. 2013.
    The effects of sleep extension on sleep and cognitive
    performance in adolescents with chronic sleep reduction: an
    experimental study. *Sleep Medicine* 14:510–7.
58 Gradisar, M., Gardner, G. & Dohnt, H. 2011. Recent
    worldwide sleep patterns and problems during adolescence: a
    review and meta-analysis of age, region, and sleep. *Sleep
    Medicine* 12:110–8.
59 Blake, M., Waloszek, J. M., Schwartz, O., et al. 2016. The
    SENSE study: post intervention effects of a randomized
    controlled trial of a cognitive-behavioral and mindfulness-
    based group sleep improvement intervention among at-risk
    adolescents. *Journal of Consulting and Clinical Psychology*
    84:1039–51.
60 Campbell, I. G. & Feinberg, I. 2009. Longitudinal trajectories
    of non-rapid eye movement delta and theta EEG as indicators
    of adolescent brain maturation. *Proceedings of the National
    Academy of Sciences of the United States of America* 106:5177–80.

61 Ohayon, M. M., Carskadon, M. A., Guilleminault, C., et al.
     2004. Meta-analysis of quantitative sleep parameters from
     childhood to old age in healthy individuals: developing
     normative sleep values across the human lifespan. *Sleep*
     27:1255–73.
62 Mednick, S. C., Christakis, N. A. & Fowler, J. H. 2010. The
     spread of sleep loss influences drug use in adolescent social
     networks. *PloS One* 5:e9775.
63 McMakin, D. L., Dahl, R. E., Buysse, D. J., et al. 2016.
     The impact of experimental sleep restriction on affective
     functioning in social and nonsocial contexts among
     adolescents. *Journal of Child Psychology and Psychiatry*
     57:1027–37.
64 Neill, F. 2015. *The Good Girl*. Penguin, London.

Chapter 5: Sleep in Youth: Sleep, Atypical Development and Mental Health

1 Paruthi, S., Brooks, L. J., D'Ambrosio, C., et al. 2016.
    Recommended amount of sleep for pediatric populations: a
    consensus statement of the American Academy of Sleep
    Medicine. *Journal of Clinical Sleep Medicine* 12:785–6.
2 Mindell, J. A. & Owens, J. A. 2015. *A Clinical Guide to
    Pediatric Sleep: Diagnosis and management of sleep problems.*
    3rd ed. Wolters Kluwer, Philadelphia.
3 Moffitt, T. E., Caspi, A., Taylor, A., et al. 2010. How
    common are common mental disorders? Evidence that
    lifetime prevalence rates are doubled by prospective versus
    retrospective ascertainment. *Psychological Medicine*
    40:899–909.
4 Merikangas, K. R., He, J. P., Burstein, M., et al. 2010.
    Lifetime prevalence of mental disorders in U.S.
    adolescents: results from the national comorbidity survey
    replication-adolescent supplement (NCS-A). *Journal of the
    American Academy of Child and Adolesccent Psychiatry*
    49:980–9.
5 Gregory, A. M. & Sadeh, A. 2016. Annual Research Review:
    sleep problems in childhood psychiatric disorders – a review
    of the latest science. *Journal of Child Psychology & Psychiatry*
    57:296–317.

6   American Psychiatric Association. 2013. *Diagnostic and Statistical Manual of Mental Disorders*. 5th ed. American Psychiatric Association, Washington, DC.

7   Willcutt, E. 2012. The prevalence of DSM-IV Attention-Deficit/Hyperactivity Disorder: a meta-analytic review. *Neurotherapeutics* 9:490–9.

8   Maris, M., Verhulst, S., Wojciechowski, M., et al. 2016. Prevalence of obstructive sleep apnea in children with Down Syndrome. *Sleep* 39:699–704.

9   Elrod, M. G. & Hood, B. S. 2015. Sleep differences among children with autism spectrum disorders and typically developing peers: a meta-analysis. *Journal of Developmental and Behavioral Pediatrics* 36:166–77.

10 Rossignol, D. A. & Frye, R. E. 2011. Melatonin in autism spectrum disorders: a systematic review and meta-analysis. *Developmental Medicine and Child Neurology* 53:783–92.

11 Dahl, R. E. 1996. The regulation of sleep and arousal: development and psychopathology. *Development and Psychopathology* 8:3–27.

12 Cha, A. E. 2017. Could some ADHD be a type of sleep disorder? That would fundamentally change how we treat it. www.washingtonpost.com/news/to-your-health/wp/2017/09/22/could-adhd-be-a-type-of-sleep-disorder-that-would-fundamentally-change-how-we-treat-it/?utm_term=.87b94cbb2f43..

13 Cortese, S. & Angriman, M. 2017. Treatment of sleep disorders in youth with ADHD: what is the evidence from randomised controlled trials and how should the field move forward? *Expert Review of Neurotherapeutics* 17:525–7.

14 Van der Heijden, K. B., Smits, M. G., Van Someren, E. J. W., et al. 2005. Idiopathic chronic sleep onset insomnia in attention–deficit/hyperactivity disorder: a circadian rhythm sleep disorder. *Chronobiology International* 22:559–70.

15 Boyce, W. T. & Ellis, B. J. 2005. Biological sensitivity to context: I. An evolutionary-developmental theory of the origins and functions of stress reactivity. *Development and Psychopathology* 17:271–301.

16 Ivanenko, A., Crabtree, V. M. & Gozal, D. 2005. Sleep and depression in children and adolescents. *Sleep Medicine Reviews* 9:115–29.

17 Haeffel, G. J. & Vargas, I. 2011. Resilience to depressive symptoms: the buffering effects of enhancing cognitive style and positive life events. *Journal of Behavior Therapy and Experimental Psychiatry* 42:13–8.

18 Gregory, A. M., Rijsdijk, F. V., Eley, T. C., et al. 2016. A longitudinal twin and sibling study of associations between insomnia and depression symptoms in young adults. *Sleep* 39:1985–92.

19 Gehrman, P. R., Meltzer, L. J., Moore, M., et al. 2011. Heritability of insomnia symptoms in youth and their relationship to depression and anxiety. *Sleep* 34:1641–6.

20 Yoo, S. S., Gujar, N., Hu, P., et al. 2007. The human emotional brain without sleep – a prefrontal amygdala disconnect. *Current Biology* 17:R877–R878.

21 Irwin, M. R., Olmstead, R. & Carroll, J. E. 2016. Sleep disturbance, sleep duration, and inflammation: a systematic review and meta-analysis of cohort studies and experimental sleep deprivation. *Biological Psychiatry*, 80:40–52

22 Lopresti, A. L., Maker, G. L., Hood, S. D., et al. 2014. A review of peripheral biomarkers in major depression: the potential of inflammatory and oxidative stress biomarkers. *Progress in Neuro-Psychopharmacology & Biological Psychiatry* 48:102–11.

23 Baumeister, D., Russell, A., Pariante, C. M., et al. 2014. Inflammatory biomarker profiles of mental disorders and their relation to clinical, social and lifestyle factors. *Social Psychiatry and Psychiatry Epidemiology* 49:841–9.

24 Urrila, A. S., Karlsson, L., Kiviruusu, O., et al. 2012. Sleep complaints among adolescent outpatients with major depressive disorder. *Sleep Medicine* 13:816–23.

25 Littlewood, D. L., Gooding, P., Kyle, S. D., et al. 2016. Understanding the role of sleep in suicide risk: qualitative interview study. *British Medical Journal Open* 6:e012113.

26 Liu, X. & Buysse, D. J. 2005. Sleep and youth suicidal behavior: a neglected field. *Current Opinion in Psychiatry* 19:288–93.

27 Alfano, C. A., Ginsburg, G. S. & Kingery, J. N. 2007. Sleep-related problems among children and adolescents with anxiety disorders. *Journal of the American Academy of Child and Adolescent Psychiatry* 46:224–32.

28 Forbes, E. E., Bertocci, M. A., Gregory. A. M., et al. 2008.
    Objective sleep in pediatric anxiety disorders and major
    depressive disorder. *Journal of the American Academy of Child
    and Adolescent Psychiatry* 47:148–55.

29 Reynolds, K. C. & Alfano, C. A. 2016. Things that go bump in
    the night: frequency and predictors of nightmares in anxious
    and nonanxious children. *Behavioral Sleep Medicine* 14:442–56.

30 Peterman, J. S., Carper, M. M. & Kendall, P. C. 2014. Anxiety
    disorders and comorbid sleep problems in school-aged youth:
    review and future research directions. *Child Psychiatry &
    Human Development* 45:1–17.

31 Chan, M. S., Chung, K. F., Yung, K. P., et al. 2017. Sleep in
    schizophrenia: a systematic review and meta-analysis of
    polysomnographic findings in case-control studies. *Sleep
    Medicine Reviews* 32:69–84.

32 Lee, Y. J., Cho, S-J., Cho, I. H., et al. 2012. The relationship
    between psychotic-like experiences and sleep disturbances in
    adolescents. *Sleep Medicine* 13:1021–7.

33 Fisher, H. L., Lereya, S. T., Thompson, A., et al. 2014.
    Childhood parasomnias and psychotic experiences at age 12
    years in a United Kingdom birth cohort. *Sleep* 37:475–82.

34 Taylor, M. J., Gregory, A. M., Freeman, D., et al. 2015. Do
    sleep disturbances and psychotic-like experiences in
    adolescence share genetic and environmental influences?
    Journal of Abnormal Psychology 124:674–84.

35 Lunsford-Avery, J. R., Orr, J. M., Gupta, T., et al. 2013.
    Sleep dysfunction and thalamic abnormalities in adolescents
    at ultra high-risk for psychosis. *Schizophrenia Research*
    151:148–53.

36 Walker, M. P. & van der Helm, E. 2009. Overnight therapy?
    The role of sleep in emotional brain processing. *Psychological
    Bulletin* 135:731–48.

37 Frick, P. J., Ray, J. V., Thornton, L. C., et al. 2014. Annual
    Research Review: a developmental psychopathology
    approach to understanding callous-unemotional traits in
    children and adolescents with serious conduct problems.
    Journal of Child Psychology and Psychiatry 55:532–48.

38 Denis, D., Akhtar, R., Holding, B. C., et al. 2017.
    Externalizing behaviors and callous-unemotional traits:
    different associations with sleep quality. *Sleep* 40: https://doi.
    org/10.1093/sleep/zsx070.

39 Poulton, R., Moffitt, T. E. & Silva, P. A. 2015. The Dunedin
    Multidisciplinary Health and Development Study: overview
    of the first 40 years, with an eye to the future. *Social
    Psychiatry and Psychiatric Epidemiology* 50:679–93.
40 Gregory, A. M., Caspi, A., Eley, T. C., et al. 2005.
    Prospective longitudinal associations between persistent
    sleep problems in childhood and anxiety and depression
    disorders in adulthood. *Journal of Abnormal Child Psychology*
    33:157–63.
41 Alvaro, P. K., Roberts, R. M. & Harris, J. K. 2013. A
    systematic review assessing bidirectionality between sleep
    disturbances, anxiety, and depression. *Sleep* 36:1059–68.
42 Freeman, D., Startup, H., Myers, E., et al. 2013. The effects
    of using cognitive behavioural therapy to improve sleep for
    patients with delusions and hallucinations (the BEST study):
    study protocol for a randomized controlled trial. *Trials*
    14:214.
43 Freeman, D., Sheaves, B., Goodwin, G. M., et al. 2017. The
    effects of improving sleep on mental health (OASIS): a
    randomised controlled trial with mediation analysis. *Lancet
    Psychiatry* 4:749–58.
44 Wolf, E., Kuhn, M., Normann, C., et al. 2016. Synaptic
    plasticity model of therapeutic sleep deprivation in major
    depression. *Sleep Medicine Reviews* 30:53–62.
45 Boland, E. M., Rao, H. Y., Dinges, D. F., et al. 2017.
    Meta-analysis of the antidepressant effects of acute sleep
    deprivation. *The Journal of Clinical Psychiatry*
    78:e1020–e1034.
46 Steinberg, H. & Hegerl, U. 2014. Johann Christian August
    Heinroth on sleep deprivation as a therapeutic option for
    depressive disorders. *Sleep Medicine* 15:1159–64.

Chapter 6: Becoming an Adult: A Sleep a Day Helps Us Work, Rest and Play

1 Hirshkowitz, M., Whiton, K., Albert, S. M., et al. 2015.
   National Sleep Foundation's sleep time duration
   recommendations: methodology and results summary. *Sleep
   Health* 1:40–3.
2 Giedd, J. N., Lalonde, F. M., Celano, M. J., et al. 2009.
   Anatomical brain magnetic resonance imaging of typically

developing children and adolescents. *Journal of the American Academy of Child and Adolescent Psychiatry* 48:465–70.

3   Lee, K. A. & Rosen, L. A. 2012. Sleep and human development. Edited by Morin, C. M. & Espie, C. A., *The Oxford Handbook of Sleep and Sleep Disorders.* Oxford University Press, Oxford. 75–94.

4   Roenneberg, T., Kuehnle, T., Pramstaller, P. P., et al. 2004. A marker for the end of adolescence. *Current Biology* 14:R1038–R1039.

5   Ohayon, M. M., Carskadon, M. A., Guilleminault, C., et al. 2004. Meta-analysis of quantitative sleep parameters from childhood to old age in healthy individuals: developing normative sleep values across the human lifespan. *Sleep* 27:1255–73.

6   Benitez, A. & Gunstad, J. 2012. Poor sleep quality diminishes cognitive functioning independent of depression and anxiety in healthy young adults. *Clinical Neuropsychologist* 26:214–23.

7   Hysing, M., Harvey, A. G., Linton, S. J., et al. 2016. Sleep and academic performance in later adolescence: results from a large population-based study. *Journal of Sleep Research* 25:318–24.

8   Hu, X. Q., Antony, J. W., Creery, J. D., et al. 2015. Unlearning implicit social biases during sleep. *Science* 348:1013–5.

9   Pilcher, J. J. & Huffcutt, A. I. 1996. Effects of sleep deprivation on performance: a meta-analysis. *Sleep* 19:318–26.

10 Dewald, J. F., Meijer, A. M., Oort, F. J., et al. 2010. The influence of sleep quality, sleep duration and sleepiness on school performance in children and adolescents: a meta-analytic review. *Sleep Medicine Reviews* 14:179–89.

11 Gregory, A. M., Caspi, A., Moffitt, T. E., et al. 2009. Sleep problems in childhood predict neuropsychological functioning in adolescence. *Pediatrics* 123:1171–6.

12 Krause, A. J., Simon, E. B., Mander, B. A., et al. 2017. The sleep-deprived human brain. *Nature Reviews Neuroscience* 18:404–18.

13 Talamas, S. N., Mavor, K. I., Axelsson, J., et al. 2016. Eyelid-openness and mouth curvature influence perceived intelligence beyond attractiveness. *Journal of Experimental Psychology-General* 145:603–20.

14 Axelsson, J., Sundelin, T., Ingre, M., et al. 2010. Beauty sleep: experimental study on the perceived health and attractiveness of sleep deprived people. *British Medical Journal* 341:c6614.

15 Oyetakin-White, P., Suggs, A., Koo, B., et al. 2015. Does poor sleep quality affect skin ageing? *Clinical and Experimental Dermatology* 40:17–22.

16 Miller, M. A., Kruisbrink, M., Wallace, J., et al. 2018. Sleep duration and incidence of obesity in infants, children and adolescents: a systematic review and meta-analysis of prospective studies. *Sleep*, https://doi.org/10.1093/sleep/zsy018.

17 Patel, S. R. & Hu, F. B. 2008. Short sleep duration and weight gain: a systematic review. *Obesity* 16:643–53.

18 Al Khatib, H. K., Harding, S. V., Darzi, J., et al. 2017. The effects of partial sleep deprivation on energy balance: a systematic review and meta-analysis. *European Journal of Clinical Nutrition* 71:614–24.

19 Greer, S. M., Goldstein, A. N. & Walker, M. P. 2013. The impact of sleep deprivation on food desire in the human brain. *Nature Communications* 4:2259.

20 Wylleman, P. & Reints, A. 2010. A lifespan perspective on the career of talented and elite athletes: perspectives on high-intensity sports. *Scandinavian Journal of Medicine & Science in Sports* 20:88–94.

21 Kredlow, M. A., Capozzoli, M. C., Hearon, B. A., et al. 2015. The effects of physical activity on sleep: a meta-analytic review. *Journal of Behavioral Medicine* 38:427–49.

22 Driver, H. S. & Taylor, S. R. 2000. Exercise and sleep. *Sleep Medicine Reviews* 4:387–402.

23 Kubitz, K. A., Landers, D. M., Petruzzello, S. J., et al. 1996. The effects of acute and chronic exercise on sleep – A meta-analytic review. *Sports Medicine* 21:277–91.

24 Brand, S., Kalak, N., Gerber, M., et al. 2014. High self-perceived exercise exertion before bedtime is associated with greater objectively assessed sleep efficiency. *Sleep Medicine* 15:1031–6.

25 Buman, M. P., Phillips, B. A., Youngstedt, S. D., et al. 2014. Does nighttime exercise really disturb sleep? Results from the 2013 National Sleep Foundation Sleep in America Poll. *Sleep Medicine* 15:755–61.

26 Chennaoui, M., Arnal, P. J., Sauvet, F., et al. 2015. Sleep and exercise: a reciprocal issue? *Sleep Medicine Reviews* 20:59–72.

27 Leeder, J., Glaister, M., Pizzoferro, K., et al. 2012. Sleep
    duration and quality in elite athletes measured using
    wristwatch actigraphy. *Journal of Sports Sciences* 30:541–5.
28 Gupta, L., Morgan, K. & Gilchrist, S. 2017. Does elite sport
    degrade sleep quality? A systematic review. *Sports Medicine*
    47:1317–33.
29 Jurimae, J., Maestu, J., Purge, P., et al. 2004. Changes in
    stress and recovery after heavy training in rowers. *Journal of
    Science and Medicine in Sport* 7:335–9.
30 VanBruggen, M. D., Hackney, A. C., McMurray, R. G.,
    et al. 2011. The relationship between serum and salivary
    cortisol levels in response to different intensities of exercise.
    International Journal of Sports Physiology and Performance
    6:396–407.
31 Fisher, S. P., Cui, N., McKillop, L. E., et al. 2016. Stereotypic
    wheel running decreases cortical activity in mice. *Nature
    Communications* 7:13138.
32 Halson, S. L. 2008. Nutrition, sleep and recovery. *European
    Journal of Sport Science* 8:119–26.
33 Foster, R. G. & Kreitzman, L. 2017. *Circadian Rhythms – A
    Very Short Introduction*. Oxford University Press, Oxford.
34 Fullagar, H. H., Duffield, R., Skorski, S., et al. 2015. Sleep
    and recovery in team sport: current sleep-related issues
    facing professional team-sport athletes. *International Journal of
    Sports Physiology and Performance* 10:950–7.
35 Gamble, J. 2016. Life in circadia. aeon.co/essays/
    soon-we-will-see-chrono-attached-to-every-form-of-
    medicine.
36 Facer-Childs, E. & Brandstaetter, R. 2015. The impact of
    circadian phenotype and time since awakening on diurnal
    performance in athletes. *Current Biology* 25:518–22.
37 Tamaki, M., Bang, J. W., Watanabe, T., et al. 2016. Night
    watch in one brain hemisphere during sleep associated
    with the first-night effect in humans. *Current Biology*
    26:1190–4.
38 Halson, S. L. 2014. Sleep in elite athletes and nutritional
    interventions to enhance sleep. *Sports Medicine* 44:13–23.
39 Bonnar, D., Bartel, K., Kakoschke, N., et al. 2018. Sleep
    interventions designed to improve athletic performance and
    recovery: a systematic review of current approaches. *Sports
    Medicine* 48:683–703.

40 Bergeron, M. F., Mountjoy, M., Armstrong, N., et al. 2015.
    International Olympic Committee consensus statement on
    youth athletic development. *British Journal of Sports Medicine*
    49:843–51.
41 McCartt, A. T., Mayhew, D. R., Braitman, K. A., et al.
    2009. Effects of age and experience on young driver crashes:
    review of recent literature. *Traffic Injury Prevention*
    10:209–19.
42 Lyznicki, J. M., Doege, T. C., Davis, R. M., et al. 1998.
    Sleepiness, driving, and motor vehicle crashes. *Journal of the
    American Medical Association* 279:1908–13.
43 Steinberg, L. 2004. Risk taking in adolescence: what
    changes, and why? *Annals of the New York Academy of Sciences*
    1021:51–8.
44 Maric, A., Montvai, E., Werth, E., et al. 2017. Insufficient
    sleep: enhanced risk-seeking relates to low local sleep
    intensity. *Annals of Neurology* 82:409–18.
45 Akerstedt, T., Kecklund, G. & Horte, L. G. 2001. Night
    driving, season, and the risk of highway accidents. *Sleep*
    24:401–6.
46 Philip, P., Sagaspe, P., Moore, N., et al. 2005. Fatigue, sleep
    restriction and driving performance. *Accident Analysis and
    Prevention* 37:473–8.
47 Watson, N. F., Morgenthaler, T., Chervin, R., et al. 2015.
    Confronting drowsy driving: the American Academy of
    Sleep Medicine Perspective. *Journal of Clinical Sleep Medicine*
    11:1335–6.
48 Horne, J. A. & Reyner, L. A. 1995. Sleep-related vehicle
    accidents. *British Medical Journal* 310:565–7.
49 Teff, B. C. 2014. Prevalence of motor vehicle crashes
    involving drowsy drivers, U.S. 2009–2013. www.newsroom.
    aaa.com/wp-content/uploads/2014/11/AAAFoundation-
    DrowsyDriving-Nov2014.pdf.

Chapter 7: Sleep During the Rush-Hour Years of Our Lives

1 Hirshkowitz, M., Whiton, K., Albert, S. M., et al. 2015.
    National Sleep Foundation's sleep time duration
    recommendations: methodology and results summary. *Sleep
    Health* 1:40–3.

2 Walch, O. J., Cochran, A. & Forger, D. B. 2016. A global quantification of 'normal' sleep schedules using smartphone data. *Science Advances* 2:e1501705.

3 Zhang, B. & Wing, Y. K. 2006. Sex differences in insomnia: a meta-analysis. *Sleep* 29:85–93.

4 Aviva UK. 2016. Nation of sleepless nights – one in four UK adults want a better night's sleep. www.aviva.co.uk/media-centre/story/17693/nation-of-sleepless-nights-one-in-four-uk-adults-w.

5 Friborg, O., Bjorvatn, B., Amponsah, B., et al. 2012. Associations between seasonal variations in day length (photoperiod), sleep timing, sleep quality and mood: a comparison between Ghana (5 degrees) and Norway (69 degrees). *Journal of Sleep Research* 21:176–84.

6 Grandner, M. A., Williams, N. J., Knutson, K. L., et al. 2016. Sleep disparity, race/ethnicity, and socioeconomic position. *Sleep Medicine* 18:7–18.

7 Mulkerrins, J. 2016. Kim Cattrall on insomnia: 'What I felt in spades was how alone I was'. www.telegraph.co.uk/women/life/kim-cattrall-on-insomnia-what-i-felt-in-spades-was-how-alone-i-w/.

8 Harvey, A. G. 2002. A cognitive model of insomnia. *Behaviour Research & Therapy* 40:869–93.

9 Espie, C. A. 2002. Insomnia: conceptual issues in the development, persistence, and treatment of sleep disorder in adults. *Annual Review of Psychology* 53:215–43.

10 Meltzer, L. J., Hiruma, L. S., Avis, K., et al. 2015. Comparison of a commercial accelerometer with polysomnography and actigraphy in children and adolescents. *Sleep* 38:1323–30.

11 Patel, P., Kim, J. Y. & Brooks, L. J. 2017. Accuracy of a smartphone application in estimating sleep in children. *Sleep and Breathing* 21:505–11.

12 Baron, K. G., Duffecy, J., Berendsen, M. A., et al. 2017. Feeling validated yet? A scoping review of the use of consumer-targeted wearable and mobile technology to measure and improve sleep. *Sleep Medicine Reviews.* www.sciencedirect.com/science/article/pii/S1087079216301496.

13 de Zambotti, M., Goldstone, A., Claudatos, S., et al. 2017. A validation study of Fitbit Charge 2 compared with

polysomnography in adults. *Chronobiology International* DOI: 10.1080/07420528.2017.1413578.

14 Riemann, D., Spiegelhalder, K., Feige, B., et al. 2010. The hyperarousal model of insomnia: a review of the concept and its evidence. *Sleep Medicine Reviews* 14:19–31.

15 Ong, J. C., Ulmer, C. S. & Manber, R. 2012. Improving sleep with mindfulness and acceptance: a metacognitive model of insomnia. *Behaviour Research & Therapy* 50:651–60.

16 Gu, J., Strauss, C., Bond, R., et al. 2015. How do mindfulness-based cognitive therapy and mindfulness-based stress reduction improve mental health and wellbeing? A systematic review and meta-analysis of mediation studies. *Clinical Psychology Review* 37:1–12.

17 Ong, J. C. & Smith, C. E. 2017. Using mindfulness for the treatment of insomnia. *Current Sleep Medicine Reports* 3:57–65.

18 Qaseem, A., Kansagara, D., Forciea, M. A., et al. 2016. Management of chronic insomnia disorder in adults: a clinical practice guideline from the American College of Physicians. *Annals of Internal Medicine* 165:125–33.

19 Blake, M., Waloszek, J. M., Schwartz, O., et al. 2016. The SENSE study: post intervention effects of a randomized controlled trial of a cognitive-behavioral and mindfulness-based group sleep improvement intervention among at-risk adolescents. *Journal of Consulting & Clinical Psychology* 84:1039–51.

20 McMakin, D. L., Siegle, G. J. & Shirk, S. R. 2011. Positive affect stimulation and sustainment (PASS) module for depressed mood: a preliminary investigation of treatment-related effects. *Cognitive Therapy and Research* 35:217–26.

21 Thiart, H., Ebert, D. D., Lehr, D., et al. 2016. Internet-based Cognitive Behavioral Therapy for Insomnia: a health economic evaluation. *Sleep* 39:1769–78.

22 Drake, C. L. 2016. The promise of digital CBT-I. *Sleep* 39:13–4.

23 Gates, P. J., Albertella, L. & Copeland, J. 2014. The effects of cannabinoid administration on sleep: a systematic review of human studies. *Sleep Medicine Reviews* 18:477–87.

24 Mehdi, T. 2012. Benzodiazepines revisited. *British Journal of Medical Practitioners* 5:a501.

25 Harmon, K. 2011. What is propofol – and how could it have killed Michael Jackson? www.scientificamerican.com/article/propofol-michael-jackson-doctor.

26 Duke, A. 2013. Expert: Michael Jackson went 60 days without real sleep. www.edition.cnn.com/2013/06/21/showbiz/jackson-death-trial/index.html?iref=allsearch.

27 Troxel, W. M., Robles, T. F., Hall, M., et al. 2007. Marital quality and the marital bed: examining the covariation between relationship quality and sleep. *Sleep Medicine Reviews* 11:389–404.

28 Morris, T. 2015. *In our Time (Circadian Rhythms)* www.bbc.co.uk/programmes/b06rzd44.

29 McArdle, N., Kingshott, R., Engleman, H. M., et al. 2011. Partners of patients with sleep apnoea/hypopnoea syndrome: effect of CPAP treatment on sleep quality and quality of life. *Thorax* 56:513–8.

30 Parish, J. M. & Lyng, P. J. 2003. Quality of life in bed partners of patients with obstructive sleep apnea or hypopnea after treatment with continuous positive airway pressure. *Chest* 124:942–7.

31 Horne, J. 2007. *Sleepfaring.* Oxford University Press, Oxford. 230–9.

32 Puhan, M. A., Suarez, A., Lo Cascio, C., et al. 2006. Didgeridoo playing as alternative treatment for obstructive sleep apnoea syndrome: randomised controlled trial. *British Medical Journal* 332:266.

33 Troxel, W. M., Braithwaite, S. R., Sandberg, J. G., et al. 2017. Does improving marital quality improve sleep? Results from a marital therapy trial. *Behavioral Sleep Medicine* 15:330–43.

34 Chen, Q., Yang, H., Zhou, N. Y., et al. 2016. Inverse U-shaped association between sleep duration and semen quality: longitudinal observational study (MARHCS) in Chongqing, China. *Sleep* 39:79–86.

35 Jensen, T. K., Andersson, A. M., Skakkebaek, N. E., et al. 2013. Association of sleep disturbances with reduced semen quality: a cross-sectional study among 953 healthy young Danish men. *American Journal of Epidemiology* 177:1027–37.

36 Kloss, J. D., Perlis, M. L., Zamzow, J. A., et al. 2015. Sleep, sleep disturbance, and fertility in women. *Sleep Medicine Reviews* 22:78–87.

37 Mindell, J. A., Cook, R. A. & Nikolovski, J. 2015. Sleep patterns and sleep disturbances across pregnancy. *Sleep Medicine* 16:483–8.

38 Hedman, C., Pohjasvaara, T., Tolonen, U., et al. 2002. Effects of pregnancy on mothers' sleep. *Sleep Medicine* 3:37–42.

39 Chang, J. J., Pien, G. W., Duntley, S. P., et al. 2010. Sleep deprivation during pregnancy and maternal and fetal outcomes: is there a relationship? *Sleep Medicine Reviews* 14:107–14.

40 August, E. M., Salihu, H. M., Biroscak, B. J., et al. 2013. Systematic review on sleep disorders and obstetric outcomes: scope of current knowledge. *American Journal of Perinatology* 30:323–34.

41 Palagini, L., Gemignani, A., Banti, S., et al. 2014. Chronic sleep loss during pregnancy as a determinant of stress: impact on pregnancy outcome. *Sleep Medicine* 15:853–9.

42 Insana, S. P. & Montgomery-Downs, H. E. 2013. Sleep and sleepiness among first-time postpartum parents: a field- and laboratory-based multimethod assessment. *Developmental Psychobiology* 55:361–72.

43 Gay, C. L., Lee, K. A. & Lee, S-Y. 2004. Sleep patterns and fatigue in new mothers and fathers. *Biological Research for Nursing* 5:311–8.

44 Malish, S., Arastu, F. & O'Brien, L. M. 2016. A preliminary study of new parents, sleep disruption, and driving: a population at risk? *Maternal and Child Health Journal* 20:290–7.

45 Doheny, K. 2017. Kids mean less sleep for mom, but not dad. www.chicagotribune.com/lifestyles/health/sc-moms-get-less-sleep-than-dads-health-0308-20170228-story.html.

46 Shockey, T. M. & Wheaton, A. G. 2017. Short sleep duration by occupation group – 29 States, 2013–2014. *Morbidity and Mortality Weekly Report* 66:7–13.

47 Nugent, C. N. & Black, L. I. 2016. Sleep duration, quality of sleep, and use of sleep medication, by sex and family type, 2013–2014. *National Centre for Health Statistics Data Brief* 230: 1–8.

48 Kahn, M., Fridenson, S., Lerer, R., et al. 2014. Effects of one night of induced night-wakings versus sleep restriction on

sustained attention and mood: a pilot study. *Sleep Medicine* 15:825–32.

49 Meltzer, L. J. & Montgomery-Downs, H. E. 2011. Sleep in the family. *Pediatric Clinics of North America* 58:765–74.

50 Hagen, E. W., Mirer, A. G., Palta, M., et al. 2013. The sleep-time cost of parenting: sleep duration and sleepiness among employed parents in the Wisconsin Sleep Cohort Study. *American Journal of Epidemiology* 177:394–401.

51 Meltzer, L. J. & Mindell, J. A. 2007. Relationship between child sleep disturbances and maternal sleep, mood and parenting stress: a pilot study. *Journal of Family Psychology* 21:67–73.

52 Gallagher, J. 2014. Night work 'throws body into chaos'. www.bbc.co.uk/news/health-25812422.

53 Coughlan, S. 2017. Sleep loss 'starts arguments at work'. www.bbc.co.uk/news/education-39444997.

54 Gowler, R. 2015. Sleep deprivation damaging business. www.hrmagazine.co.uk/article-details/sleep-deprivation-damaging-business.

55 Bramoweth, A. D. & Germain, A. 2013. Deployment-related insomnia in military personnel and veterans. *Current Psychiatry Reports* 15:401, https://doi.org/10.1007/s11920-013-0401-4.

56 Barger, L. K., Flynn-Evans, E. E., Kubey, A., et al. 2014. Prevalence of sleep deficiency and use of hypnotic drugs in astronauts before, during, and after spaceflight: an observational study. *Lancet Neurology* 13:904–12.

57 Philips, T. 2014. Wide awake on the sea of tranquility. www.nasa.gov/exploration/home/19jul_seaoftranquillity.html.

58 Dawson, D. & Reid, K. 1997. Fatigue, alcohol and performance impairment. *Nature* 388:235.

59 Stain, S. C. & Farquhar, M. 2017. Should doctors work 24-hour shifts? *British Medical Journal* 358:j3522.

60 Kennedy, M. 2013. Moritz Erhardt death: intern's parents feared he was exhausted at work. www.theguardian.com/business/2013/nov/22/moritz-erhadt-death-exhaustion-parents-bank-america-epilepsy..

61 Shahly, V., Berglund, P. A., Coulouvrat, C., et al. 2012. The associations of insomnia with costly workplace accidents and errors results from the America Insomnia Survey. *Archives of General Psychiatry* 69:1054–63.

62 Huffpost. 2013. Five other disastrous accidents related to
    sleep deprivation. www.huffingtonpost.com/2013/12/03/
    sleep-deprivation-accidents-disasters_n_4380349.html.

63 Hafner, M., Stepanek, M., Taylor, J., et al. 2016. Why sleep
    matters – the economic costs of insufficient sleep: a cross-
    country comparative analysis. Santa Monica, California,
    USA: RAND Ciroiratuib.

64 Dinges, D. F., Pack, F., Williams, K., et al. 1997. Cumulative
    sleepiness, mood disturbance, and psychomotor vigilance
    performance decrements during a week of sleep restricted to
    4–5 hours per night. *Sleep* 20:267–77.

65 von Bonsdorff, M. B., Strandberg, A., von Bonsdorff, M.,
    et al. 2017. Working hours and sleep duration in midlife as
    determinants of health-related quality of life among older
    businessmen. *Age and Ageing* 46:108–12.

66 Vogel, M., Braungardt, T., Meyer, W., et al. 2012. The
    effects of shift work on physical and mental health. *Journal of
    Neural Transmission* 119:1121–32.

67 Wang, F., Yeung, K., Chan, W., et al. 2013. A meta-
    analysis on dose-response relationship between night shift
    work and the risk of breast cancer. *Annals of Oncology*
    24:2724–32.

68 Wang, X., Ji, A., Zhu, Y., et al. 2015. A meta-analysis
    including dose-response relationship between night shift
    work and the risk of colorectal cancer. *Oncotarget*
    6:25046–60.

69 Gan, Y., Yang, C., Tong, X., et al. 2015. Shift work and
    diabetes mellitus: a meta-analysis of observational studies.
    Occupational and Environmental Medicine 72:72–78.

70 Vyas, M. V., Garg, A. X., Iansavichus, A. V., et al. 2012. Shift
    work and vascular events: systematic review and meta-
    analysis. *British Medical Journal* 345:e4800.

71 Van Dycke, K. C., Rodenburg, W., van Oostrom, C. T.,
    et al. 2015. Chronically alternating light cycles increase
    breast cancer risk in mice. *Current Biology* 25:1932–7.

72 Roenneberg, T. & Merrow, M. 2016. The circadian clock
    and human health. *Current Biology* 26:R432–R443.

73 Travis, R. C., Balkwill, A., Fensom, G. K., et al. 2016. Night
    shift work and breast cancer incidence: three prospective
    studies and meta-analysis of published studies. *Journal of the
    National Cancer Institute* 108:djw169.

74 Stevens, R. G. 2017. Night shift work and breast cancer incidence: three prospective studies and meta-analysis of published studies. *Journal of the National Cancer Institute* 109:djw342.

75 Dibner, C., Schibler, U. & Albrecht, U. 2010. The mammalian circadian timing system: organization and coordination of central and peripheral clocks. *Annual Review of Physiology* 72:517–49.

76 Akerstedt, T. 2003. Shift work and disturbed sleep/wakefulness. *Occupational Medicine* 53:89–94.

77 Saksvik, I. B., Bjorvatn, B., Hetland, H., et al. 2011. Individual differences in tolerance to shift work – A systematic review. *Sleep Medicine Reviews* 15:221–35.

78 Short, M. A., Agostini, A., Lushington, K., et al. 2015. A systematic review of the sleep, sleepiness, and performance implications of limited wake shift work schedules. *Scandinavian Journal of Work Environment & Health* 41:425–40.

79 Henry, Z. 2015. Six companies (including Uber) where it's OK to nap. www.inc.com/zoe-henry/google-uber-and-other-companies-where-you-can-nap-at-the-office.html.

80 Hafner, M. & Troxel, W. M. 2016. How business can take the lead in getting people to sleep more. http://journal.thriveglobal.com/businesses-can-take-the-lead-in-getting-people-to-sleep-more-ab0d18f472a5.

81 Silverberg, D. 2016. The company that pays its staff to sleep. www.bbc.co.uk/news/business-36641119.

82 Viola, A. U., James, L. M., Schlangen, L. J. M., et al. 2008. Blue-enriched white light in the workplace improves self-reported alertness, performance and sleep quality. *Scandinavian Journal of Work Environment & Health* 34:297–306.

Chapter 8: It's a Long Hard Night: The Sleep of Older Adults

1 Hirshkowitz, M., Whiton, K., Albert, S. M., et al. 2015. National Sleep Foundation's sleep time duration recommendations: methodology and results summary. *Sleep Health* 1:40–3.

2 2015. Olive Cooke inquest: Poppy seller suffered depression. www.bbc.co.uk/news/uk-england-bristol-33550581.

3 Samson, D. R., Crittenden, A. N., Mabulla, I. A., et al. 2017. Chronotype variation drives night-time sentinel-like behaviour in hunter-gatherers. *Proceedings of the Royal Society B-Biological Sciences* 284:20170967.

4 Ohayon, M. M., Carskadon, M. A., Guilleminault, C., et al. 2004. Meta-analysis of quantitative sleep parameters from childhood to old age in healthy individuals: developing normative sleep values across the human lifespan. *Sleep* 27:1255–73.

5 Crowley, K. 2011. Sleep and sleep disorders in older adults. *Neuropsychology Review* 21:41–53.

6 Zdanys, K. F. & Steffens, D. C. 2015. Sleep disturbances in the elderly. *Psychiatric Clinics of North America* 38:723–41.

7 Vaughan, C. P. & Bliwise, D. L. 2018. Sleep and nocturia in older adults. *Sleep Medicine Clinics* 13:107–16.

8 Cornu, J. N., Abrams, P., Chapple, C. R., et al. 2012. A contemporary assessment of nocturia: definition, epidemiology, pathophysiology, and management – a systematic review and meta-analysis. *European Urology* 62:877–90.

9 Redden, S. 2013. Older workers statistical information booklet. *Official Statistics.*

10 Foley, D. J., Monjan, A. A., Brown, S. L., et al. G. 1995. Sleep complaints among elderly persons – an epidemiologic-study of 3 communities. *Sleep* 18:425–32.

11 Lim, A. S. P., Ellison, B. A., Wang, J. L., et al. 2014. Sleep is related to neuron numbers in the ventrolateral preoptic/intermediate nucleus in older adults with and without Alzheimer's disease. *Brain* 137:2847–61.

12 Cohen-Mansfield, J., Hazan, H., Lerman, Y., et al. 2016. Correlates and predictors of loneliness in older-adults: a review of quantitative results informed by qualitative insights. *International Psychogeriatrics* 28:557–76.

13 Hawkley, L. C. & Cacioppo, J. T. 2010. Loneliness matters: a theoretical and empirical review of consequences and mechanisms. *Annals of Behavioral Medicine* 40:218–27.

14 Matthews, T., Danese, A., Gregory, A. M., et al. 2017. Sleeping with one eye open: loneliness and sleep quality in young adults. *Psychological Medicine* 47:2177–86.

15 Shaver, J. L. & Woods, N. F. 2015. Sleep and menopause: a narrative review. *Menopause* 22:899915.

16 Vahratian, A. 2017. Sleep duration and quality among women
    aged 40-59, by menopausal status. www.cdc.gov/nchs/data/
    databriefs/db286.pdf.

17 Lockley, S. W. & Foster, R. G. 2012. Sleep: a very short
    introduction. Oxford University Press, Oxford.

18 Salvi, S. M., Akhtar, S. & Currie, Z. 2006. Ageing changes
    in the eye. *Postgraduate Medical Journal* 82:581–7.

19 Ayaki, M., Muramatsu, M., Negishi, K., et al. 2013.
    Improvements in sleep quality and gait speed after cataract
    surgery. *Rejuvenation Research* 16:35–42.

20 Potter, V. 2017. *Patient H69: The Story of My Second Sight.*
    Bloomsbury, London.

21 Auld, F., Maschauer, E. L., Morrison, I., et al. 2017. Evidence
    for the efficacy of melatonin in the treatment of primary
    adult sleep disorders. *Sleep Medicine Reviews* 34:10–22.

22 Milic, J., Saavedra Perez, H., Zuurbier, L. A., et al. 2017. The
    longitudinal and cross-sectional associations of grief and
    complicated grief with sleep quality in older adults.
    Behavioral Sleep Medicine. https://doi.org/10.1080/15402002.2
    016.1276016.

23 Willis, T. A., Yearall, S. M. & Gregory, A. M. 2011. Self-
    reported sleep quality and cognitive style in older adults.
    Cognitive Therapy and Research 35:1–10.

24 Smagula, S. F., Stone, K. L., Fabio, A., et al. 2016. Risk
    factors for sleep disturbances in older adults: evidence from
    prospective studies. *Sleep Medicine Reviews* 25:21–30.

25 Duffy, J. F., Willson, H. J., Wang, W., et al. 2009. Healthy
    older adults better tolerate sleep deprivation than young
    adults. *Journal of the American Geriatrics Society* 57:1245–51.

26 Jackowska, M., Hamer, M., Carvalho, L. A., et al. 2012.
    Short sleep duration is associated with shorter telomere
    length in healthy men: findings from the Whitehall II
    Cohort Study. *PloS One* 7:e47292.

27 James, S., McLanahan, S., Brooks-Gunn, J., et al. 2017. Sleep
    duration and telomere length in children. *Journal of Pediatrics*
    187:247–52.

28 Nobelprize.org. 2018. Average age of Nobel Laureates in all
    prize categories. www.nobelprize.org/nobel_prizes/lists/
    laureates_ages/all_ages.html.

29 Lo, J. C., Groeger, J. A., Cheng, G. H., et al. 2016. Self-
    reported sleep duration and cognitive performance in older

adults: a systematic review and meta-analysis. *Sleep Medicine* 17:87–98.

30   Holth, J. K., Patel, T. K. & Holtzman, D. M. 2017. Sleep in Alzheimer's disease – beyond amyloid. *Neurobiology of Sleep and Circadian Rhythms* 2:4–14.

31   Sveinbjornsdottir, S. 2016. The clinical symptoms of Parkinson's disease. *Journal of Neurochemistry* 139:318–24.

32   Schenck, C. H., Boeve, B. F. & Mahowald, M. W. 2013. Delayed emergence of a parkinsonian disorder or dementia in 81% of older men initially diagnosed with idiopathic rapid eye movement sleep behavior disorder: a 16-year update on a previously reported series. *Sleep Medicine* 14:744–8.

33   Musiek, E. S. & Holtzman, D. M. 2016. Mechanisms linking circadian clocks, sleep, and neurodegeneration. *Science* 354:1004–8.

34   Shan, Z. L., Ma, H. F., Xie, M. L., et al. 2015. Sleep duration and risk of type 2 diabetes: a meta-analysis of prospective studies. *Diabetes care* 38:529–37.

35   Cappuccio, F. P., Cooper, D., D'Elia, L., et al. 2011. Sleep duration predicts cardiovascular outcomes: a systematic review and meta-analysis of prospective studies. *European Heart Journal* 32:1484–92.

36   King, C. R., Knutson, K. L., Rathouz, P. J., et al. 2008. Short sleep duration and incident coronary artery calcification. *Journal of the American Medical Association* 300:2859–66.

37   Shahar, E., Whitney, C. W., Redline, S., et al. 2001. Sleep-disordered breathing and cardiovascular disease: cross-sectional results of the sleep heart health study. *American Journal of Respiratory and Critical Care Medicine* 163:19–25.

38   Hla, K. M., Young, T., Hagen, E. W., et al. 2015. Coronary heart disease incidence in sleep disordered breathing: the Wisconsin Sleep Cohort Study. *Sleep* 38:677–84.

39   Erren, T. C., Morfeld, P., Foster, R. G., et al. 2016. Sleep and cancer: synthesis of experimental data and meta-analyses of cancer incidence among some 1,500,000 study individuals in 13 countries. *Chronobiology International* 33:325–50.

40   Shantha, G. P. S., Kumar, A. A., Cheskin, L. J., et al. 2015. Association between sleep-disordered breathing, obstructive sleep apnea, and cancer incidence: a systematic review and meta-analysis. *Sleep Medicine* 16:1289–94.

41   Nieto, F. J., Peppard, P. E., Young, T., et al. 2012. Sleep-
     disordered breathing and cancer mortality results from the
     Wisconsin sleep cohort study. *American Journal of Respiratory
     and Critical Care Medicine* 186:190–4.

42   Almendros, I., Montserrat, J. M., Ramirez, J., et al. 2012.
     Intermittent hypoxia enhances cancer progression in a mouse
     model of sleep apnoea. *European Respiratory Journal* 39:215–7.

43   Prather, A. A., Janicki-Deverts, D., Hall, M. H., et al. 2015.
     Behaviorally assessed sleep and susceptibility to the common
     cold. *Sleep* 38:1353–9.

44   Irwin, M. R., Wang, M., Ribeiro, D., et al. 2008. Sleep loss
     activates cellular inflammatory signaling. *Biological Psychiatry*
     64:538–40.

45   Frighetto, L., Marra, C., Bandali, S., et al. 2004. An
     assessment of quality of sleep and the use of drugs with
     sedating properties in hospitalized adult patients. *Health and
     Quality of Life Outcomes* 2:17.

46   Griffiths, M. F. & Peerson, A. 2005. Risk factors for chronic
     insomnia following hospitalization. *Journal of Advanced
     Nursing* 49:245–53.

47   Tamrat, R., Huynh-Le, M. P. & Goyal, M. 2014.
     Non-pharmacologic interventions to improve the sleep of
     hospitalized patients: a systematic review. *Journal of General
     Internal Medicine* 29:788–95.

48   Schrimpf, M., Liegl, G., Boeckle, M., et al. 2015. The effect
     of sleep deprivation on pain perception in healthy subjects: a
     meta-analysis. *Sleep Medicine* 16:1313–20.

49   Kaur, G., Phillips, C., Wong, K., et al. 2013. Timing is
     important in medication administration: a timely review of
     chronotherapy research. *International Journal of Clinical
     Pharmacy* 35:344–58.

50   Long, J. E., Drayson, M. T., Taylor, A. E., et al. 2016.
     Morning vaccination enhances antibody response over
     afternoon vaccination: a cluster-randomised trial. *Vaccine*
     34:2679–85.

51   Dew, M. A., Hoch, C. C., Buysse, D. J., et al. 2003. Healthy
     older adults' sleep predicts all-cause mortality at 4 to 19 years
     of follow-up. *Psychosomatic Medicine* 65:63–73.

52   Cappuccio, F. P., D'Elia, L., Strazzullo, P., et al. 2010. Sleep
     duration and all-cause mortality: a systematic review and
     meta-analysis of prospective studies. *Sleep* 33:585–92.

53 Liu, T. Z., Xu, C., Rota, M., et al. 2017. Sleep duration and
    risk of all-cause mortality: a flexible, non-linear, meta-
    regression of 40 prospective cohort studies. *Sleep Medicine
    Reviews* 32:28–36.
54 Itani, O., Jike, M., Watanabe, N. & Kaneita, Y. 2017. Short
    sleep duration and health outcomes: a systematic review,
    meta-analysis, and meta-regression. *Sleep Medicine* 32:246–56.
55 Jike, M., Itani, O., Watanabe, N., et al. 2017. Long sleep
    duration and health outcomes: a systematic review, meta-
    analysis and meta-regression. *Sleep Medicine Reviews*. www.
    sciencedirect.com/science/article/pii/S1087079217300278.
56 Mitler, M. M., Hajdukovic, R. M., Shafor, R., et al. 1987.
    When people die – cause of death versus time of death.
    American Journal of Medicine 82:266–74.
57 Smolensky, M. H., Portaluppi, F., Manfredini, R., et al.
    2015. Diurnal and twenty-four-hour patterning of human
    diseases: cardiac, vascular, and respiratory diseases,
    conditions, and syndromes. *Sleep Medicine Reviews* 21:3–11.

Chapter 9: A Ticket to the Land of Nod: Tips to Get Your Best Sleep and Make Dreams Come True

1 Hirshkowitz, M., Whiton, K., Albert, S. M., et al. 2014.
   National Sleep Foundation's sleep time duration
   recommendations: methodology and results summary. *Sleep
   Health* 1:40–3.
2 Rodgers, P. 2014. The sleep deprivation epidemic. www.
   forbes.com/sites/paulrodgers/2014/09/09/
   the-sleep-deprivation-epidemic/#7982f81cb897.
3 Ford, E. S., Cunningham, T. J. & Croft, J. B. 2015. Trends in
   self-reported sleep duration among US adults from 1985 to
   2012. *Sleep* 38:829–32.
4 National Sleep Foundation. 2006. Sleep in America poll.
   sleepfoundation.org/sites/default/files/2006_summary_of_
   findings.pdf.
5 Yetish, G., Kaplan, H., Gurven, M., et al. 2015. Natural sleep
   and its seasonal variations in three pre-industrial societies.
   Current Biology 25:2862–8.
6 Kronholm, E., Partonen, T., Laatikainen, T., et al. 2008.
   Trends in self-reported sleep duration and insomnia-related
   symptoms in Finland from 1972 to 2005: a comparative

review and re-analysis of Finnish population samples. *Journal of Sleep Research* 17:54–62.

7   Keyes, K. M., Maslowsky, J., Hamilton, A., et al. 2015. The great sleep recession: changes in sleep duration among US adolescents, 1991–2012. *Pediatrics* 135:460–8.

8   Matricciani, L., Olds, T. & Petkov, J. 2012. In search of lost sleep: secular trends in the sleep time of school-aged children and adolescents. *Sleep Medicine Reviews* 16:203–11.

9   Youngstedt, S. D., Goff, E. E., Reynolds, A. M., et al. 2016. Has adult sleep duration declined over the last 50+years? *Sleep Medicine Reviews* 28:69–85.

10   Knutson, K. L., Van Cauter, E., Rathouz, P. J., et al. 2010. Trends in the prevalence of short sleepers in the USA: 1975–2006. *Sleep* 33:37–45.

11   Ekirch, A. R. 2005. *At Day's Close*. Weidenfeld & Nicolson, London.

12   Ekirch, A. R. 2016. Segmented sleep in preindustrial societies. *Sleep* 39:715–6.

13   Bauters, F., Rietzschel, E. R., Hertegonne, K. B. C., et al. 2016. The link between obstructive sleep apnea and cardiovascular disease. *Current Atherosclerosis Reports* 18:1 https://doi.org/10.1007/s11883-015-0556-z.

14   Vaessen, T. J. A., Overeem, S. & Sitskoorn, M. M. 2015. Cognitive complaints in obstructive sleep apnea. *Sleep Medicine Reviews* 19:51–8.

15   Garbarino, S., Guglielmi, O., Sanna, A., et al. 2016. Risk of occupational accidents in workers with obstructive sleep apnea: systematic review and meta-analysis. *Sleep* 39:1211–8.

16   *Telegraph* Reporters. Carrie Fisher died from sleep apnea and a combination of other factors, coroner concludes. www.telegraph.co.uk/films/2017/06/17/carrie-fisher-died-sleep-apnea-combination-factors-coroner-concludes/.

17   Marsh, R. & Shortell, D. 2016. NJ train engineer in crash had undiagnosed sleep apnoea. edition.cnn.com/2016/11/17/us/njt-engineer-sleep-apnea/index.html.

18   Gill, I. & McBrien, J. 2017. Effectiveness of melatonin in treating sleep problems in children with intellectual disability. *Archives of Disease in Childhood* 102:870–3.

19   Kennaway, D. J. 2015. Potential safety issues in the use of the hormone melatonin in paediatrics. *Journal of Paediatrics and Child Health* 51:584–9.

20 Qaseem, A., Kansagara, D., Forciea, M. A., et al. 2016. Management of chronic insomnia disorder in adults: a clinical practice guideline from the American College of Physicians. *Annals of Internal Medicine* 165:125–33.
21 Schlarb, A. A., Bihlmaier, I., Velten-Schurian, K., et al. 2016. Short- and long-term effects of CBT-I in groups for school-age children suffering from chronic insomnia: the KiSS-program. *Behavioral Sleep Medicine* https://doi.org/10.1080/15402002.2016.1228642.
22 Eichenwald, E. C. 2016. Apnea of prematurity. *Pediatrics* 137:e20153757.
23 Clark, I. & Landolt, H. P. 2017. Coffee, caffeine, and sleep: a systematic review of epidemiological studies and randomized controlled trials. *Sleep Medicine Reviews* 31:70–8.
24 Drake, C., Roehrs, T., Shambroom, J., et al. 2013. Caffeine effects on sleep taken 0, 3, or 6 hours before going to bed. *Journal of Clinical Sleep Medicine* 9:1195–200.
25 Ebrahim, I. O., Shapiro, C. M., Williams, A. J., et al. 2013. Alcohol and sleep I: effects on normal sleep. *Alcoholism: Clinical and Experimental Research* 37:539–49.
26 Chan, J. K., Trinder, J., Colrain, I. M., et al. 2015. The acute effects of alcohol on sleep electroencephalogram power spectra in late adolescence. *Alcoholism: Clinical and Experimental Research* 39:291–9.
27 Grandner, M. A., Kripke, D. F., Naidoo, N., et al. 2010. Relationships among dietary nutrients and subjective sleep, objective sleep, and napping in women. *Sleep Medicine* 11:180–4.
28 Cao, Y., Wittert, G., Taylor, A. W., et al. 2016. Associations between macronutrient intake and obstructive sleep apnoea as well as self-reported sleep symptoms: results from a cohort of community dwelling Australian men. *Nutrients* 8:207.
29 Lauer, C. J. & Krieg, J. C. 2004. Sleep in eating disorders. *Sleep Medicine Reviews* 8:109–18.
30 St-Onge, M. P., Mikic, A. & Pietrolungo, C. E. 2016. Effects of diet on sleep quality. *Advances in Nutrition* 7:938–49.
31 Wehrens, S. M. T., Christou, S., Isherwood, C., et al. 2017. Meal timing regulates the human circadian system. *Current Biology* 27:1768–75.e3.
32 de la Pena, I. J., Hong, E., de la Pena, J. B., et al. 2015. Milk collected at night induces sedative and anxiolytic-like effects and augments pentobarbital-induced sleeping behavior in mice. *Journal of Medicinal Food* 18:1255–61.

33 Feng, X. Y., Wang, M., Zhao, Y. Y., et al. 2014. Melatonin
    from different fruit sources, functional roles, and analytical
    methods. *Trends in Food Science & Technology* 37:21–31.

34 Howatson, G., Bell, P. G., Tallent, J., et al. 2012. Effect of
    tart cherry juice (Prunus cerasus) on melatonin levels and
    enhanced sleep quality. *European Journal of Nutrition*
    51:909–16.

35 Kim, J., Lee, S. L., Kang, I., et al. 2018. Natural products
    from single plants as sleep aids: a systematic review. *Journal of
    Medicinal Food* https://doi.org/10.1089/jmf.2017.4064.

36 Fernandez-San-Martin, I. M., Masa-Font, R., Palacios-Soler,
    L., et al. 2010. Effectiveness of Valerian on insomnia: A
    meta-analysis of randomized placebo-controlled trials. *Sleep
    Medicine* 11:505–11.

37 Faraut, B., Andrillon, T., Vecchierini, M. F., et al. 2017.
    Napping: a public health issue. From epidemiological to
    laboratory studies. *Sleep Medicine Reviews* 35:85–100.

38 Hilditch, C. J., Dorrian, J. & Banks, S. 2017. A review of
    short naps and sleep inertia: do naps of 30 min or less really
    avoid sleep inertia and slow-wave sleep? *Sleep Medicine*
    32:176–90.

39 Kim, E-J. & Dimsdale, J. E. 2007. The effect of psychosocial
    stress on sleep: a review of polysomnographic evidence.
    Behavioral Sleep Medicine 5:256–78.

40 Meston, C. M. & Buss, D. M. 2007. Why humans have sex.
    Archives of Sexual Behavior 36:477–507.

41 Mah, K. & Binik, Y. M. 2001. The nature of human orgasm:
    a critical review of major trends. *Clinical Psychology Review*
    21:823–56.

42 Wang, C. F., Sun, Y. L. & Zang, H. X. 2014. Music therapy
    improves sleep quality in acute and chronic sleep disorders: a
    meta-analysis of 10 randomized studies. *International Journal of
    Nursing Studies* 51:51–62.

43 Bei, B., Wiley, J. F., Trinder, J., et al. 2016. Beyond the
    mean: a systematic review on the correlates of daily
    intraindividual variability of sleep/wake patterns. *Sleep
    Medicine Reviews* 28:108–24.

44 Ross, J. J. 1965. Neurological findings after prolonged sleep
    deprivation. *Archives of Neurology* 12:399–403.

45 Gulevich, G., Dement, W. & Johnson, L. 1966. Psychiatric
    and EEG observations on a case of prolonged (264 hours)
    wakefulness. *Archives of General Psychiatry* 15:29–35.

46 Walch, O. J., Cochran, A. & Forger, D. B. 2016. A global quantification of 'normal' sleep schedules using smartphone data. *Science Advances* 2:e1501705.

47 Gangwisch, J. E., Babiss, L. A., Malaspina, D., et al. 2010. Earlier parental set bedtimes as a protective factor against depression and suicidal ideation. *Sleep* 33:97–106.

48 Stothard, E. R., Mchill, A. W., Depner, C. M., et al. 2017. Circadian entrainment to the natural light-dark cycle across seasons and the weekend. *Current Biology* 27:508–13.

49 Leung, C. & Ge, H. 2013. Sleep thermal comfort and the energy saving potential due to reduced indoor operative temperature during sleep. *Building and Environment* 59:91–8.

50 Moon, R. Y., Darnall, R. A., Feldman-Winter, L., et al. 2016. SIDS and other sleep-related infant deaths: evidence base for 2016 updated recommendations for a safe infant sleeping environment. *Pediatrics* 138:e20162940.

51 Krauchi, K. 2007. The thermophysiological cascade leading to sleep initiation in relation to phase of entrainment. *Sleep Medicine Reviews* 11:439–51.

52 Obradovich, N., Migliorini, R., Mednick, S. C., et al. 2017. Night-time temperature and human sleep loss in a changing climate. *Science Advances* 3:e1601555.

53 American Academy of Sleep Medicine. Sleep or Netflix? You can have both when you binge-watch responsibly. www.aasm.org/sleep-or-netflix-you-can-have-both-when-you-binge-watch-responsibly.

54 Boor, B. E., Spilak, M. P., Laverge, J., et al. 2017. Human exposure to indoor air pollutants in sleep microenvironments: a literature review. *Building and Environment* 125:528–55.

55 National Sleep Foundation. 2011. Bedroom Poll: summary of findings. www.sleepfoundation.org/sites/default/files/bedroompoll/NSF_Bedroom_Poll_Report.pdf.

56 Tischer, C., Chen, C. M. & Heinrich, J. 2011. Association between domestic mould and mould components, and asthma and allergy in children: a systematic review. *European Respiratory Journal* 38:812–24.

57 Tiesler, C. M. T., Thiering, E., Tischer, C., et al. 2015. Exposure to visible mould or dampness at home and sleep problems in children: results from the LISAplus study. *Environmental Research* 137:357–63.

58 Strom-Tejsen, P., Zukowska, D., Wargocki, P., et al. 2016.
    The effects of bedroom air quality on sleep and next-day
    performance. *Indoor Air* 26:679–86.
59 Krahn, L. E., Tovar, M. D. & Miller, B. 2015. Are pets in the
    bedroom a problem? *Mayo Clinic Proceedings* 90:1663–5.
60 Patel, S. I., Miller, B. W., Kosiorek, H. E., et al. 2017. The
    effect of dogs on human sleep in the home sleep
    environment. *Mayo Clinic Proceedings* 92:1368–72.
61 Ohayon, M., Wickwire, E. M., Hirshkowitz, M., et al. 2017.
    National Sleep Foundation's sleep quality recommendations:
    first report. *Sleep Health* 3:6–19.
62 Harvey, A. G. 2002. A cognitive model of insomnia.
    Behaviour Research & Therapy 40:869–93.
63 Hertenstein, E., Thiel, N., Luking, M., et al. 2014. Quality
    of life improvements after acceptance and commitment
    therapy in nonresponders to cognitive behavioral therapy for
    primary insomnia. *Psychotherapy and Psychosomatics* 83:371–3.
64 Saunders, D. T., Roe, C. A., Smith, G., et al. 2016. Lucid
    dreaming incidence: a quality effects meta-analysis of 50
    years of research. *Consciousness and Cognition* 43:197–215.
65 Hobson, A. 2009. The neurobiology of consciousness: lucid
    dreaming wakes up. *International Journal of Dream Research* 2:41–4.
66 Stumbrys, T., Erlacher, D., Schadlich, M., et al. 2012.
    Induction of lucid dreams: a systematic review of evidence.
    Consciousness and Cognition 21:1456–75.
67 Smith, B. V. & Blagrove, M. 2015. Lucid dreaming frequency
    and alarm clock snooze button use. *Dreaming* 25:291–9.
68 Murillo-Rodriguez, E., Barciela Versa, A., Barbosa Rocha,
    N., et al. 2017. An overview of the clinical uses,
    pharmacology, and safety of modafinil. *ACS Chemical
    Neuroscience*: https://doi.org/10.1021/acschemneuro.7b00374
69 Battleday, R. M. & Brem, A. K. 2015. Modafinil for cognitive
    neuroenhancement in healthy non-sleep-deprived subjects: a
    systematic review. *European Neuropsychopharmacology* 25:1865–81.
70 Chivers, T. 2013. How much do we really know about sleep?
    www.telegraph.co.uk/news/science/10494965/How-much-
    do-we-really-know-about-sleep.html.
71 Horne, J. 2007. *Sleepfaring*. Oxford University Press, Oxford.

Acknowledgements

First and foremost, thank you to my boys Hector and Orson for their endless energy – but equally for agreeing to sleep once in a while so I could work on this book. To my beloved husband, The Golden Wolf (AKA Paul Taylor) – I'm grateful for everything, but perhaps most of all my daily zeitgeber of coffee in bed. To my parents Joanna and Gerry Gregory, for no doubt allowing me to disrupt your sleep regularly throughout the years.

Thanks to Jim Martin, Bloomsbury publisher and friend, who proved that he was far from a 1980s executive, by 'getting' the importance of sleep straight away. I am also grateful to Anna MacDiarmid for her input and support throughout and to my excellent copy editor Emily Kearns. Thanks also to the superb illustrator Marc Dando. I have a lot to thank the other Bloomsbury authors for too, including Rob Brotherton, Liam Drew, Vanessa Potter, Laurie Winkless and Helen Scales – and to the additional members of Neuwrite including Roma Agrawal and Christine Dixon.

A particular thanks to the many sleep experts for their generous input – whether providing feedback, quotes, flagging additional interesting articles or for their general kindness. Their help has been truly invaluable, however any errors in the text are all mine. These experts include Daniel Buysse, Erika Forbes, Lisa Meltzer, Brian Sharpless, Sarah Blunden, Malcolm von Schantz, Brant Hasler, Michael Grandner, Michael Gradisar, Roger Ekirch, Stephanie Crowley-McWilliam, Luci Wiggs, Kristin Knutson, Jason Ong, Nicola Barclay, Dan Denis, Megan Crawford, Colin Espie, Simon Archer, Mike Parsons, Dieter Riemann, Candice Alfano, Peter Franzen, Rotem Perach, Sibah Hassan, Wendy Troxel and Kira Vibe Jespersen.

Other academics have also provided invaluable support or feedback, including my dear friend Essi Viding, as well as Ian Craig, Tim Matthews, Louise Arseneault, Angelica Ronald, Tom O'Connor, Lucy Foulkes, Jon Mill, Chloe Wong and

Richard Rowe. Thanks too to the many academics who have made a huge difference to my career, including Allison Harvey for introducing me to sleep research; Avi Sadeh, wonderful collaborator and friend whose inspiration and advice I miss so greatly; and Thalia Eley, Avshalom Caspi and Temi Moffitt who have been my main mentors, supporting me throughout my career – becoming both role models and friends. I am also incredibly grateful to the many students and collaborators who have taught me so much – and whose work I have described in this book.

Thanks also to my beloved family and friends for sharing their excitement about this project. There are too many to name all here – but a few stand out, including Mary Anderson-Ford for breezily renaming this book *Nodding Off*, reading two drafts, and her friendship and enthusiasm throughout. James Smithies was incredibly supportive, entertaining my kids and offering his time and expertise. He kindly read every chapter multiple times, despite this not being a classics book. Thanks also to Rashad Braimah and Gabriele Esu for their kindness and tips along the way. Thanks too to my sister Anna Gregory for commenting on an early draft and to her husband Joe Shrapnel. Thanks to Christy Kirkpatrick for her inside publishing knowledge and tips, as well as her friendship. I am also grateful to Ed Fitzhugh, Nick Raggett, Lynne Huby, Esther Paterson, Ali Newport, Ciara McEwen, Bryony Weale, Joanne Jensen, Ed Horrox, Adriana Martyr, Gerry Girou, Maria Napolitano, Nizar El-Chamaa, Rachel Jupp, Rebecca Mitchell, Jenny Stock, Kitty Travers, Hiroe Baba and Ana Richmond. Thanks to Grandma and Grandpa 'The Heap' for (together with my parents) looking after my wolf pups, allowing me to write this book.

I am grateful to my friends and colleagues at Goldsmiths. In particular to Chris French for convincing me not to give up at any of the various hurdles (and for being an excellent luncheon companion). He also read the entire book and has given support throughout. I'm also particularly grateful to Yulia Kovas, Lauren Stewart, Caspar Addyman and Gustav Kuhn who have read early chapters or sections of this book. And Joydeep Bhattacharya for his feedback on the Figure.

Thanks to the many special children in my life: my nephews Holden and Harlan, as well as Felix, Andre, William, Harry, Toby and Baby Alice.

Finally, to the countless people who have allowed me to include their own experiences and anecdotes (anonymised) in this book: I am immensely grateful and wish you lots of restful sleep in the years ahead.

Index